TANTRIC
SEX
AND
MENOPAUSE

"Through a wide range of methods and tools, the authors offer practical advice to support your health and emotional well-being during menopause. By releasing old disempowering beliefs, dropping tired and worn-out expectations, allowing yourself to express emotions healthfully, and putting yourself and your needs first, they offer a holistic, supportive paradigm to nourish your body and soul, to honor yourself and your partner, to experience real intimacy and deep love on a level previously unimaginable. They invite you to come home to the wisdom, power, and truth of who you are."

BRANDON BAYS, INTERNATIONALLY BESTSELLING AUTHOR
OF *THE JOURNEY* AND *FREEDOM IS*

"The journey of embodiment has been life changing for me. Thank you, Diana and Janet, for writing this book while I embrace menopause. I could not ask for a better guidebook. This work in the realm of sexuality is truly groundbreaking and opens up a magnificent realm of possibility and fulfillment hitherto unimaginable."

CATHERINE OXENBERG, ACTRESS, AUTHOR,
PRODUCER, AND PHILANTHROPIST

"An uplifting and empowering read. The authors have shared so much wisdom and demystified so many myths—it's astounding!! This book offers inspiring stories from women with open hearts and courageous souls and many great tips and practices to access your own knowing and body wisdom. I feel this book is for women of all ages to read and create a new collective voice of what menopause and intimacy can be."

VANESSA FINNIGAN, EDITOR AND PUBLISHER OF
HOLISTIC BLISS MAGAZINE

"Through its simple, yet elegant, practices and empowering information, *Tantric Sex and Menopause* is an inspiring guide that gives the power back to women through this transition, while still honoring men. It will speak to all women, no matter what age, who wish to truly understand femininity and the journey of womanhood at its core. I was inspired and uplifted by this heart-opening book."

RACHAEL JAYNE GROOVER, AUTHOR OF *POWERFUL AND FEMININE* AND CREATOR OF ART OF FEMININE PRESENCE™

"A woman's midlife rebirth is a revolutionary passage that we're only just beginning to honor. We are urgently in need of the wise council and fierce love of seasoned experts in feminine embodiment like Diana Richardson and Janet McGeever to show us that, far from being the end, menopause should be celebrated as a glorious new awakening. This is the book we've been waiting for."

LISA SCHRADER, AUTHOR OF *KAMA SUTRA 52*, COACH, AND FOUNDER OF AWAKENINGSHAKTI.COM

"*Tantric Sex and Menopause* offers great help to menopausal women and couples who wish to continue to be sexual and grow in their lovemaking. Thank you to authors Diana Richardson and Janet McGeever for sharing such practical and beneficial wisdom. May it help many people!"

MERCEDES KIRKEL, AUTHOR OF *SUBLIME UNION: A WOMAN'S SEXUAL ODYSSEY GUIDED BY MARY MAGDALENE*

"This is the book women need most right now. Whether you are peri- or postmenopausal, this book gives the gift of empowerment. It is high time that women in middle age and beyond are embraced as the multifaceted sexual beings they are. *Tantric Sex and Menopause* does just that and more."

SUZANNA MILLER, BLOGGER AND PODCASTER AT BLISSRUNNER.COM

"*Tantric Sex and Menopause* opens the door and introduces a new way of being sexual that is nurturing to the feminine body. I was struck by the empathy for the journey of women and felt a deep sense of support and connection within this book. It offers a recalibration of a woman's sexuality, emotional health, and understanding of menopause. This book is full of hormone and body knowledge and practices that empower. I love this book."

MARY SPICER, LIFE SOLUTIONS COACH, ENERGY MEDICINE PRACTITIONER, AND RADIO HOST

TANTRIC SEX
AND
MENOPAUSE

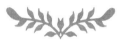

PRACTICES FOR SPIRITUAL AND SEXUAL RENEWAL

DIANA RICHARDSON
AND JANET McGEEVER

Destiny Books
Rochester, Vermont • Toronto, Canada

Destiny Books
One Park Street
Rochester, Vermont 05767
www.DestinyBooks.com

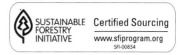

Text stock is SFI certified

Destiny Books is a division of Inner Traditions International

Library of Congress Cataloging-in-Publication Data

Names: Richardson, Diana, author. | McGeever, Janet, 1961– author.
Title: Tantric sex and menopause : practices for spiritual and sexual renewal / Diana Richardson and Janet McGeever.
Description: Rochester, Vermont : Destiny Books, [2018] | Includes bibliographical references.
Identifiers: LCCN 2017039009 (print) | LCCN 2018003707 (e-book) | ISBN 9781620556832 (paperback) | ISBN 9781620556849 (e-book)
Subjects: LCSH: Menopause—Popular works. | Middle-aged women—Sexual behavior. | Sex instruction for women. | Female orgasm. | Sex—Religious aspects—Tantrism. | BISAC: HEALTH & FITNESS / Women's Health. | SELF-HELP / Sexual Instruction.
Classification: LCC HQ46 .R466 2018 (print) | LCC HQ46 (e-book) | DDC 613.9/6—dc23
LC record available at https://lccn.loc.gov/2017039009

Printed and bound in the United States by Lake Book Manufacturing, Inc.
The text stock is SFI certified. The Sustainable Forestry Initiative® program promotes sustainable forest management.

10   9   8   7   6   5   4   3   2   1

Text design and layout by Virginia Scott Bowman
This book was typeset in Garamond Premier Pro, Avenir, and Gill Sans with Hypatia Sans and Trend Sans used as the display typefaces.
Artwork by David Andor, www.wavesourcedesign.com

"Self-Massage of Lymph System near Chest and Breasts" on pages 104–5 used by permission from Christiane Northrup, M.D., www.drnorthrup.com

To send correspondence to the authors of this book, mail a first-class letter to the authors c/o Inner Traditions • Bear & Company, One Park Street, Rochester, VT 05767, and we will forward the communication, or contact the authors directly at **www.livinglove.com** for Diana Richardson and **www.janetmcgeever.com** for Janet McGeever.

◇◇◇

To all women, past, present, and future.

Contents

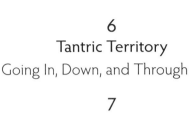

Acknowledgments

TO THE MANY COURAGEOUS WOMEN who have stepped forward on this journey, our gratitude to each and every one of you for sharing your experiences, which have served both to inspire us and to confirm our own experiences. Our heartfelt thanks also to your men, without whose presence and willingness the whole experiment in love could not be made manifest, and to the men closest to us, Michael and Gene, through and with whom we have learned and experienced an inestimable amount. Our sincere thanks for their research, resources, and inspiration to Dr. Christiane Northrup and the late Leslie Kenton, who sadly passed away just as we finished writing this book, as well as Melissa Borich, mindfulness and yoga teacher who inspired the inclusion of the yoga in this book; and Andrea Lopez for her inspiring work on Mayan abdominal healing. Many thanks also to Yollana Shore for her support and to David Andor for his cooperation in redrawing some previously published pictures, and for drawing several new ones. Last but not least, to the spiritual masters Osho and Barry Long, we offer everlasting gratitude for life-changing insights into human sexuality that revolutionized our own personal lives.

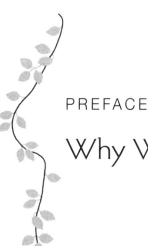

Why We Wrote This Book

OUR BOOK IS AN ENDEAVOR to shed light on the true nature of your body, and to give hope where there may be a sense of loss or little inspiration. There are many books on menopause, but few approach sex and menopause through the window of Tantra. We have both personally explored Tantra in our own relationships, and we both teach Making Love Retreats for couples, where we present an approach to sex that is life changing. And, of course, as women we have had our own unique menopause experiences, which have been very different from each other but shared many similarities.

Additionally, we have interacted with hundreds of participants (women and men) over a span of many years who have given us a wealth of direct feedback, some offered verbally and some very apparent. The impact of a tantric approach on the body and mind is undeniable: it imparts a new sense of self, a serene inner connection with the body, and a profound understanding of sex and its function beyond reproduction.

Of necessity, there will be a certain level of repetition in the chapters ahead, partly due to the interweaving themes but also to aid readers who may not read in sequence, preferring to dive into chapters randomly and independent of one another.

OUR PERSONAL BACKGROUNDS

Although women share many common elements of lovemaking and menopause, each woman's path is unique. We are both grateful that our paths intersected.

Diana: I made a conscious choice not to have children in this lifetime, a decision that was very clear for me by age thirteen. I have never questioned or regretted my decision, and I recognize in hindsight that it opened the way for me to give birth on another level—to a more profound understanding of ancient sexual knowledge and wisdom, freshly conceived and conveyed. In my early thirties I had the urge to somehow change the way I made love, and so, based on information and inspiration from tantric masters Osho in India and Barry Long in Australia—to whom I am eternally grateful—I embarked on an inquiry into sex. Essentially it was a step into the unknown, one that unwittingly propelled my life in unforeseen directions.

I had initially qualified as a lawyer in 1977 during the apartheid era in South Africa, in the hopes of being able "to be of use" in my distressed and unjust homeland. However, after six years at university, and duly graduated, I soon realized that nothing I could offer would make a drop of difference. So instead I turned to massage, intentionally opting for a life of touch and the heart in place of one that involved thinking and revolving around in my mind. So, with my aspirations for a legal career over, I followed my hands and went to the UK where I learned therapeutic massage. Over the years I also studied several other bodywork approaches. As a result I have joyfully given countless massages and taught different forms of bodywork to many hundreds of students. Thus my life has evolved in a way in which I have been fully engaged with my own body and with the bodies of other people. All that I have felt, learned, seen, and experienced through this has formed the ongoing backdrop to my sexual exploration and has shaped my understanding and perception of the body in foundational ways.

The journey has been (and still is, decades later) an unfolding undirected experience of attempting to live and love while anchored in the body (rather than circling around it) and relaxing into being and sensing (instead of getting distanced by the mind and relentless thinking). In essence I cultivated engaging my awareness (mindfulness) *via the body* in all given situations. It was and is a process of remembrance that imparts a sweetness that permeates and embraces each day. What I could not know when I began the process is that the ongoing thread of awareness and presence within the body would turn out to be a vital force that is powerfully healing, integrating, and transforming. Thus my life changed radically, yet gradually, and in ways I could not have imagined, solely through changing the way I made love—nothing more, yet nothing less.

As a by-product of my journey, in 1993 I started teaching weeklong retreats for couples, sharing my own experiences, and then in 1996 I began experimenting with whether the written word could convey the field and feelings of subtle energetic realities. This seemed to resonate with readers right from the outset, and has been extremely reassuring and encouraging. One book led to another in the intervening years, and much to my surprise, this is my eighth book. I am deeply indebted to Janet, my coauthor on this book, for her passionate collaboration, and feel honored to be working with someone of her caliber, talent, and competence.

We formed an immediate bond several years ago when Janet came to Switzerland to participate in a Making Love Retreat, and she is now an authorized teacher of the process in Australia. This means Janet is able to share from the perspective of her own experience and personal transformation via the Making Love approach, which made a vital contribution to her own menopause journey. Her fertile combination of being grounded in the Making Love approach and having a great deal to contribute regarding menopause gave rise to our collaboration.

My own menopause transition was very smooth, in the sense that I scarcely noticed it or even thought about it, much less consulted a doctor or talked with anyone about it. I cannot say why my menopause was easy—perhaps it was changing the way I made love when I was thirty, not having children, focusing on body awareness and relaxation (including thousands of massages), or having lucky genes and a light-hearted, loving mother—but because it happened by itself and I was not in any way engaged, I was unable to write from my own direct experience, as I had in my previous books.

Nevertheless, what I have learned through changing the way I make love has shaped my life on all levels, including my perceptions about menopause. Through my work teaching couples over the last twenty-five years I have ascertained that a high percentage of women find that conscious sex (rather than mechanical sex) can relieve and sometimes even heal many menopause symptoms. Beyond the physical relief, the addition of a fresh level of body awareness and mindfulness dramatically increases levels of self-worth and self-love. Many women reading this book in their forties and fifties may have a concern that it's too late to do something, but I beg you please not to give up so readily. It's worth the attempt. The body is with you, waiting for your cooperation and awareness. The spirit you embody is eternally young and fresh. How you relate to your body and "feel into" your body can have an impact on your life in a myriad of powerful, mysterious ways.

For guidance along the way, in addition to this current book I can offer you several previous books on the tantric approach, two written with my partner Michael, exploring it from different perspectives: *The Heart of Tantric Sex, Slow Sex, Tantric Orgasm for Women,* and *Tantric Sex for Men* are suggested for further reference. All of my writings describe a congruent sexual approach, presented here within the framework of menopause. While the book *Tantric Love: Feeling versus Emotion* does not explicitly deal with sex, it gives fresh insights into the potentially disruptive area of emotions and offers practical guidelines on how to manage this challenging aspect of relationships. Publishing information on all of these can be found in the recommended books section at the back of the book.

Janet: I went through an early menopause before being introduced to the Making Love approach. When I was growing up in Australia in the 1960s and '70s, my mother practiced yoga, used natural therapies and home remedies, and passed on books about the female body, all of which strongly influenced me through my late teens and early twenties. In the late '50s and early '60s, at a time when medical intervention was beginning to emerge in childbirth, my mother consciously sought a doctor who was an advocate of natural childbirth for all three of her children. Naturally dedicated to following in her path, and without even a second thought, at age twenty-three, pregnant with my first child, I also sought natural childbirth. By the time I was with my second child, at thirty (and looking back now as a mature woman), the liberating experience of giving birth at home changed me forever. This truly sparked my passion about women and our female bodies. Having experienced that profoundly instinctive and empowering journey, I had become so much more attuned and sensitive to my body that I felt I could no longer continue to have sex in the same way, even though I did compromise on many occasions. Not knowing any alternative planted a seed of questioning and created great stress for my relationship and my body, which exacerbated my other stresses of parenting and running businesses. By my mid-thirties I was chronically fatigued.

I'm forever grateful for Diana breezing into my life in the form of Australian writer Ruth Ostrow, who interviewed her in 2002 and wrote about her work for her column in *The Australian* newspaper. Just a few key words sparked hope that there was another way to make love. This launched me on a quest for something more. My immediate reaction was, *I want to meet this woman!*

Fast forward six years to forty-seven years of age when I was blessed to experience the Making Love Retreat in Switzerland, in a new relationship with a loving man for whom I am eternally grateful. Making love in relaxation changed my life and, over time, changed who I am. I believe it changed and healed the very cells of my body on a profound level, including any lingering injury or trauma from my past.

This approach to lovemaking and sexuality was what I had been searching for all my adult years. Diana's work gave me permission to appreciate being female and all that entails as a woman, mother, and now grandmother . . . and permission to trust my own instincts when it came to sex. However, because I struggled with a busy Western lifestyle in my earlier years while mothering, including long-term stress, I did experience a difficult menopause, not knowing why at the time, nor where or whom to turn to. I do wonder, if I had these tools and information at a younger age, if I could have changed the course of my menopause, at least to some degree. But the past is in the past, and in the present I am inspired to share this beautiful approach to loving and sexuality, to help other couples of all ages change the way they make love through teaching the Making Love Retreat in Australia as well as women's retreats, and through my one-to-one psychotherapy practice.

Growing up with a strict religious background, I am often completely astounded that I have ended up here. This teaching has allowed me to shed those cultural imprints to some degree and bring sexuality back to its intrinsic natural innocence—a deeply healing journey. One woman freed of her sexual conditioning creates a profound ripple that touches the heart of every person she meets, including the generations before and after her. That is my hope for you. I am sincerely grateful and forever humbled for the synchronicity of events that led to this collaboration with Diana.

Making Love through Midlife and Beyond

PERHAPS FOR THE FIRST TIME IN HISTORY, with the wave of the Baby Boomer generation (the demographic group born during the post–World War II baby boom, approximately 1946 through 1964), women are breaking new ground in many areas, in ways that were mostly unavailable to their mothers for various reasons. Many are gearing up for new careers, earning more school credits and degrees, taking greater interest in health and self-care, and even starting to value the notion of aging gracefully. This includes a fulfilling love life and sexual expression that embraces all that a woman is.

Yet in the Western world, menopause remains largely unspoken despite myriad books on the subject, and its impact on a healthy and spiritually integrated sex life even less so. This leaves women feeling isolated and inept in their perceived inability to maintain their spiritual/sexual center in these uncharted waters. We want to take menopause and our sexuality as women out from beneath the cone of silence and shine the light of tantric intelligence on it. Everything changes for a woman at this time of her life—the physical, mental, emotional, and spiritual levels are all affected.

One of the most common themes among women in their forties, fifties, and sixties, as the symptoms of perimenopause and menopause approach, is that they can begin to feel somehow sexually deficient. Sex is often no longer of interest. The thought of having sex turns them off, rather than arousing them. Sex hurts. Sex is boring. Sex is duty. Sex is pressure. Sex is to please their man. And although they may not have enjoyed unwanted stares and attention directed their way in earlier years, they now feel sexually invisible. Quite easily women feel they are discarded, washed up, cast aside, or disregarded.

While a high percentage of women do have difficulties in sex, and often well before the onset of menopause, there are women for whom this is not a problem at all and who have happily moved through lives in which sex has been fulfilling, joyous, and life enhancing. In fact, some are more sexually assertive and demanding of their men to "step up," be a "real" man, or "do the job." They may be looking for hot, lusty, superficial sex with no sharing or intimacy, and yet on the inside have a longing for love.

The advertising and fashion industries, and pornography that promotes sensational, aggressive sex, put enormous expectation and pressure on women (as well as men) of all ages, and this tension is causing an even greater rift between the sexes. By the time a woman reaches the age of fifty or sixty, if she has been in a long-term relationship, often she has given up hope. The widespread feelings of despondency, confusion, and emotional pain for both women and men are a result of the lack of constructive information that views human sexuality at a deeper level—at a level that supports, respects, and honors a woman's body and acknowledges that the female body is designed physically and energetically "equal yet opposite" to that of the male body. This is essentially the foundation of Tantra, as will be clarified in due course.

This vital difference in our body energies, beyond the physical, is groundbreaking information. Usually in sex we treat ourselves, male and female, as being more or less the same. Our culture in some ways has caused this, and so we have gone to great lengths to prove women are not "the weaker sex." However, for thousands of years there has been significant hidden knowledge pertaining to male/female energies as an interplay of dynamic and receptive forces that is largely undiscovered. These golden nuggets of knowledge now need to find their place in the modern world, whether in the East or the West, because the misunderstanding about the deeper implications of sex is global, and in some cases has had catastrophic consequences.

One of the purposes of the information in the chapters ahead is to encourage each woman with the reassurance that there is nothing inherently wrong with you as a woman, or with your body, or with your sexual reactions and responses. For our long-term health and well-being it is high time we create a crack in the powerful misconceptions around menopause and making love, so that as individuals and collectively we can begin to feel renewed strength and hope as we grow older.

In bringing this information forth we sincerely hope to empower you to claim your own body, for yourself first and foremost, and then explore what that means in the sexual exchange if you have a partner. For single women the information has equal value. Our guidance is based on the understanding that "it" is all happening within you as an individual anyway! Whether you are with a partner or not, ultimately a new vision will support you to take ownership of your own sexuality and well-being.

Allow yourself to go on a journey as you read, and to be open beyond the facts and problems of menopause to the possibilities and gifts the transition can bring. These words are an offering for you to create your own experience of menopause as you read. This could be the manual you didn't get, as the information about sex and spiritual energy was mostly unavailable to women for generations.

Our shared hope is that this book will be useful for women of all ages, including younger women currently fully engaged in their careers, long-term relationships, parenting, and so forth, who are passionate about care of their bodies and womanhood. Our understanding is that everyone, women and men alike, can learn from these pages and be encouraged by the possibilities that lie in store. Having another view can bring about a new confidence in being a woman and inspiration about the incredible privilege it is to have been born female at this time.

It is also our hope that each generation of women moving forward from here can have the information within these pages, in order to empower as many women as possible around the globe to live and experience a menopause that is as pain-free and as symptom-free as possible, especially in relation to their sexuality. We would hope that as you grow to your elder years you feel confident to pass on this information to your friends and to the younger women in your family or social circle. As we learn to accept, love, and honor our own female bodies and their extraordinary capabilities, including the wisdom lying therein, we naturally bring about peace within our hearts and relationships. This way we become messengers of peace and love for our families and our communities.

HETEROSEXUALITY AND HOMOSEXUALITY

The Making Love approach we speak of throughout this book is primarily a heterosexual teaching. However, we do not intend to exclude our lesbian sisters, and many of the principles and guidelines contained in these pages can successfully be applied to same-sex relationships. We are all women. We all bleed. We are all of our mothers' wombs. We all feel. And we all go through this transition eventually. So we welcome women of all races, creeds, gender preferences, and ages as we embark on our journey into something we all yearn for: love and its place in the context of sexual exchange, through and beyond our midlife years.

Just as we were completing this book, an email arrived from a young woman of thirty-six years who, after three years of integrating a tantric approach based on one of Diana's earlier books, told us the following story.

A New Way of Life

Your book gave me my power, my knowledge about my body, my self-determination, and my sole responsibility back. I finally had tools to change not my partner but me, my body awareness, my behaviors, my thoughts. This was the beginning of understanding sexual energy. It was the starting point of a new way of life.

It is our hope that the following pages will offer a starting point for you for a new way of life.

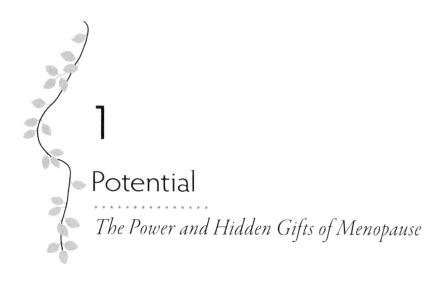

1

Potential

. . . .

The Power and Hidden Gifts of Menopause

*In Celtic cultures, the young maiden was seen as the flower;
the mother, the fruit; and the elder woman, the seed. The
seed is the part that contains the knowledge and potential
of all the other parts within it.*

CHRISTIANE NORTHRUP, M.D., *WOMEN'S BODIES,
WOMEN'S WISDOM*

THROUGH THIS POETIC AND PROFOUND description we are
absorbed into a world where the role and presence of the elder woman
was revered, respected, and held value. It was a world in which a woman
was nurtured through the next stage by her elders with love, reassurance, wisdom, and encouragement to go inward, to rest deeply within,
to sense the wellspring of her spirit and intuitive knowing; to feel herself from within her being. By contrast, a Westernized woman today is
faced with a constant focus on the outer world and the way it perceives
her, and a barrage of imagery and information telling her to be younger,
look younger, and avoid as much as possible the process of aging. She
needs to have grown up or somehow become immersed in cultures that
value *all* the stages of womanhood in order for her to naturally feel her
innate worth at this time.

One such culture is the Maya, whose traditions provide very specific care for a woman's body from girlhood onward through menstruation, pregnancy, birthing, mothering, and beyond. In Western culture, when it comes to life transitions for both men and women, we are lost in ignorance. In so many traditions and indigenous societies, and in much of our past genetic heritage, the knowledge of the body and what happens along the way is passed on with far more grace and insight than in ours. Instead we find our information in books and on the internet, never really knowing what or whom to believe or trust in the flood of information available to us, which is often tainted by a medical patriarchal mindset.

However, the silence that our forebears may have lived through around this transition is being broken, and that's definitely a good thing, but it is exceedingly common in the Western world that women are still not equipped with enough knowledge or support to move through menopause with more ease. As a culture we handle the menopause transition in a way very similar to the way we handle the onset of menstruation in earlier life, where there is typically very little support for the young girl moving into womanhood.

As women our bodies have a tremendous impact on our daily lives through menstruation, pregnancy, birthing, motherhood, and then menopause, in a way that men do not experience. All of these transitions change a woman, and if she listens deeply, the transition of menopause can carry profound wisdom that seems to simply arise within her—intuitive wisdom that can inform, transform, and cherish. It can change a woman's psyche, inviting her into her own awakening. Hot flashes (or flushes) can be seen not only as annoying occurrences but as a phenomenon in the body to be inquired into and be curious about. Therefore, menopause can be a powerful and transformational doorway ushering her into the next stage of a woman's life.

Yet tragically, the modern medical model and society in general puts the aging woman on the shelf. Men her age are sometimes looking for younger women and her self-esteem gets a battering, while at the same time she is expected to be all for everyone—including in the bedroom—and she may never really feel as if she is living up to that. Many women have passed through the intense mothering phase or have simply arrived at a stage where they don't feel able to continue living the way they have been.

In this situation a woman can evaluate the known risks and opt to make minimal adjustments. Or she may see the potential rewards and find a new resolve to increasingly honor her body more, to not compromise anymore—sexually or in family, work, or friendships—and consciously make a shift. Sometimes such a step means the end of a relationship or marriage, or at least it may precipitate upheaval. It may mean finding a new purpose, reinventing herself, or moving into her later-life's calling, sharing more of her creative gifts. She may feel called to be in more active service in her community or as a grandparent. Not least of all, she may experience a new awakening in her sexuality. Some women find that their lives improve immensely after menopause, that they are happier, healthier, and enjoy a fulfilling sex life. They often have a new and irreverent boldness to say what they think and do what they want. The bold one replaces the "good girl" as she begins to make more choices that please her, instead of always pleasing others. She becomes less willing to make excuses or compromises for others. By this time, women who have allowed others to step over their boundaries, violate them, cross them, and perhaps walk all over them seem to draw a line in the sand. It's as if their hormones are calling to them to stand up, step up, and show up in a way that was never before apparent. A welcome and incredibly empowering bonus is that she can now make love without any possibility or fear of becoming pregnant.

However, for others clearly it's a very different story. Some women feel quite broken and emotionally distraught during menopause, and carry a deep lack of self-worth, shame, even self-hatred, for not living up to the expectations of society, peers, family, or even self. Without adequate support, a woman may flounder and fall into depression and anxiety and can shut down on the emotional, physical, and sexual levels.

In the privacy of her own company, a woman may despair at the sight of her skin that was once beautiful, supple, and glowing and is now showing signs of age. Women are social creatures who generally value connecting. The separation within families, each living in separate homes cut off from others, leaves some women feeling isolated and unfulfilled. Women can easily slip through the social cracks at this stage, and sometimes develop illnesses, gain unwanted weight, or have a myriad of health issues.

At this time women need to be together to support and nurture one another, to acknowledge and strengthen each other. A woman who is more supported, informed, and aware of her potential and the potency of this phase of her life can rise through it like a phoenix that empowers the next stage.

This is the life phase in which a woman who has followed society's mandates by rote has the potential to awaken to her own self. She is being called to dig deeper than the identity of wife, partner, mother, or profession to find something that can continually sustain and nourish her from within throughout her mature years.

Menopause Life Expectancy

An estimated 6,000 U.S. women reach menopause every day (more than 2 million a year). With a life expectancy in the Western world estimated at 79.7 years, a woman who reaches the age of 54 can now reasonably expect to live to at least the age of 84, barring an unforeseen health crisis or accident.*

---

*Source: www.menopause.org.

WOMEN'S LONGEST LIFE PHASE

Given the statistics in the box above, at least one-third of a woman's life on earth will be spent as a menopausal woman, and for some it will be half her life. In a world that gives little value to the aging population, where youthfulness is a multibillion-dollar business, the prospect of moving through the change of life may never have been more daunting or disheartening than it is now. Women are constantly besieged by imagery in the media suggesting that youth is to be worshipped and aging is to be feared. Due to increased means of communication and prolonged lifespan, we are the first civilization to be confronted with this kind of "aging phenomenon." Yet, as noted above, for those who move with ease through menopause, this is a substantial amount of time in which to develop and celebrate a personal renaissance.

Beyond Society's Limitations

Again, more than ever previously, women are being called to redefine themselves beyond the lens of advertising, and beyond the lens of our social and sexual conditioning. Somehow women need to bridge the gap to this next stage of life if they are to be happy, empowered, and inspired. Somehow they must make meaning of their lives to go beyond society's limitations.

Loss of Interest in Sex

While some report feeling freed from the fears of pregnancy, many menopausal women find that the desire for intimacy simply has become nonexistent—they groan at the mention of the word *sex,* and feel resigned to the fact that sex as they know it is no longer satisfying. Sex has become "less important," yet they may still experience stress in their relationship. Could this stress possibly be the unacknowledged sexual tensions, hurts, and disappointments that can occur between man and woman? Or possibly a loud call from her psyche and body begging her to question whether the conventional way of making love still works for her?

Often a strong voice begins to call out in relation to sex. Through menopause a woman can begin to find her own voice and listen to a deeper one calling from inside. "Not this again . . ." If her pattern has been to please man, which is a very deep imprinting in all women, then her internal radar system is on high alert by this time, telling her *No more!*

But she is often flailing to find a solution because her heart still yearns for the intimacy of relationship, yet her body may not go where it used to go with conventional sex. She may feel herself in a double bind because in so many relationships, sex is the gel that has brought a couple together intimately, yet now sex is the very thing that makes her feel more and more separate, driving her away from the very one she wants to love. In a way the aching love inside her just can't get out, it can't find a passage. Her emotions can at times become overwhelming and uncontrollable and her hormones may wreak havoc on her beautiful body.

WHY TANTRA WORKS
FOR MENOPAUSAL WOMEN

Through a more informed approach to sex and beginning to access the true source of her sexual vitality and its potential, a woman can open to herself again. The symptoms that up to 75 percent of women experience around menopause—loss of interest in sex/intimacy, dryness, thinning vaginal walls, pain, anxiety, and so on—can be a surprising doorway into the incredibly gentle and relaxing world of the tantric approach to her own body as an individual . . . and if she has a partner, to a more relaxed and more conscious way of making love.

In addition, and not only when she is moving through menopause, for a woman to see that she is an equal yet opposite force to man, complementary and not subsidiary to him, can be a welcome relief. Metaphorically, the power or force that went into the body's creation of eggs is now able to lie dormant, not to atrophy, shrink, and die, but to harness the truth of sex for higher means. At any time in a woman's life, again not just in menopause, shifting her awareness to a tantric, mindful approach allows her to experience sex as a generative, enlivening force, not as a depleting, painful, or obligatory act. Instead of creating life for another, she finds she can begin to generate more life for herself.

The tantric Making Love approach that we both practice and teach offers the possibility of a long and lasting love affair with your own body and with your lover (if you have one), allowing you to step into the realm of cultivating your own sensual vitality and inner presence. Tantric sex, sometimes called "slow sex," is a beautiful bridge for a couple who are reaching their midlife years and starting to feel inevitable changes in their bodies. It's a time when heartfelt negotiation and communication between man and woman is important. Man can be welcomed into the world of sensitive awareness and, if he is open, he can discover a whole field of love and relaxation—one that brings release from what potentially can be a deeply concerning and disheartening pressure of sexual performance. No longer does he need to be working so hard at sex, getting it right. Instead the body and the genitals can be the guides. This is a welcome relief for both men and women.

Pain during Intercourse

Pain is frequently experienced during sex by women of all ages. For a woman who has had pain in the past yet still gone ahead with sex, there may be lot of tension and resistance to sex built into the tissues of her vagina, and indeed her whole body and psyche. In more sensitive and informed sex, in a safe environment, a woman is given more time and space for a true opening and awakening in the body. Along with the use of natural lubricant (see chapter 8), it allows a woman to relax more deeply into herself. She has space to be with her body on the inside, and perhaps find herself accessing something that may have been lost along the way—her exquisite internal feminine energies. The fragrance of love can suddenly become released, set free while making slow, sensual love.

With the common complaint around menopause of never really feeling ready for sex and experiencing vaginal dryness and pain, a slower, more conscious style of lovemaking gives her body more time to warm up. She is able to bring more awareness to her breasts as the energy-raising pole in her body, allowing her to come to a place of physical readiness, which in turn completely transforms her experience.

Often the cause of vaginal pain is threefold: First, a woman's vagina at rest is not energetically ready to receive, the door is not yet truly open. Second, a man on entering into the vagina may push his penis into her body, with very little awareness in the penis itself, or of the way he is using it. His focus is more on "getting in there" as quickly as possible rather than on feeling his way gradually into the canal. This push makes the connection very physical, with no energy or awareness component, and thus is likely to cause pain. As soon as a man becomes more conscious of what he is doing and how, the ensuing slowness and sensitivity will relate to and communicate with the vaginal tissues, which in turn will relax and yield more easily. So in a high percentage of cases where there is pain, there is definitely a possibility to create a big shift in experience, as elaborated in chapters 8 and 9. The third cause of pain, as discussed in more detail in the next chapter, is lower levels of estrogen in the menopausal woman's body that naturally cause a thinning of the vaginal walls, which makes them more sensitive to abrasion and discomfort.

Alternately, for the woman who has no problems or challenges moving into lovemaking during menopause, the pace of a slower style of sex opens her to sensual frontiers perhaps not previously felt. She finds her body is more joyful than ever and she freely allows and relaxes into pleasure.

Friction in the Vagina

For women who do suffer from pain during sex, a conscious approach also implies a need for less friction caused by excessive movement of the penis inside the vagina, which can be the cause of the pain in the first place. Pain also disturbs the vagina generally, making it more contracted and narrow, whereas with relaxation and awareness, the cells of the vaginal wall and indeed the whole pelvic area have time to soften and expand, readying to invite and receive a penis that becomes a welcome guest, rather than an invader and inflictor of pain.

One woman shares her story:

For the last ten years, my husband and I haven't had sex and our intimacy involved cuddling and mutual masturbation. We decided to attend the retreat and within three days I was having my husband's penis inside me comfortably— even feeling great—for the first time in over ten years. I now have a deeper relationship with my husband through having a new paradigm for approaching love, not just sex.

Expanding into Sensitivity

As menopause can invite you to greater depth and more honesty as a woman, slowness in sex is also something you can integrate into your lovemaking at any stage. If you are already naturally sensitive and more attuned than most, being more conscious can help you become even more attuned. It's an ongoing circle of awareness and attunement. A tantric approach to lovemaking enables deep insights to be harvested in the psyche. Instead of being identified with the idea of aging, or of love outside of ourselves, it enables us to feel our bodies from the inside. There is a growing feeling that our bodies work perfectly in a beautiful, harmonious, divine way. It enables us to move through our days and open to pleasure freshly, using the senses as doorways. A menopausal body is pleading: Slow down! Be more receptive, more sensitive, more conscious!

Expanding into sensitivity heralds the sacredness of love, transformation, and a deep healing of earlier years in which life may have propelled us in unwanted directions. A shift in attitude can bring a newfound centering and trust in ourselves and our deepest body truths, which allow us to have more influence in sex—to steer it in the direction of love, presence, and awareness instead of being mechanical and focused on sensation rather than sensitivity.

Menopause is an individual quest or heroine's journey for each woman to find her own way armed with knowledge, information, and her intuition and deepened connection with her body. Then she can navigate her own path to power. But this is not "power over," it is a power within—one that can move mountains. This is the true power of woman. And this journey is not outward; it is an *inward* journey.

The menopause years invite a woman to become her own person—to leave the shackles of past identification of who she is, of her roles, and transform into an expression as unique and individual as she is, of presence and love. If a woman is on track she will grow increasingly more loving and more compassionate.

Like any journey, menopause changes you. It is an undeniable gateway—a threshold. As the process is usually a gradual one, it's a slow unfolding, of initiation, of emerging. It is the grand walk into her elder years, "the second spring" as the Chinese refer to it. Menopause can potentially be a phase where a woman's sexual expression matures into something else, something deeper and more profound. There is no going back. This is the great power and potential of this incredible phase of your life.

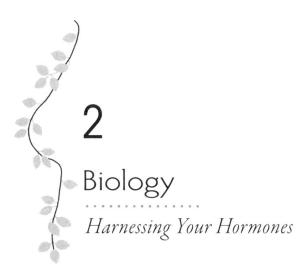

2

Biology

Harnessing Your Hormones

MANY WOMEN KNOW VERY LITTLE ABOUT the hormones in our female bodies. It's actually quite complicated so it is no wonder, and it is not the purpose of this book to go into the intricate workings of our hormones. However, we will give a general overview of what happens, as it is extremely interesting. What we do know about menopause is that our menstrual cycle changes, but it does not only mean irregular menses. The fascinating thing is that menopause involves every system of our bodies—not only the intelligent endocrine system, that is, the system that produces and regulates hormones, but also the digestive system, immune system, and nervous system.

The term *menopause* is commonly used to describe any of the changes a woman experiences either just before or after she stops menstruating, marking the end of her reproductive period and fertility. It can take approximately a ten-year span of many shifts and changes in the body. It is found that 15 percent of women have biochemistry that deals with the changes easily, and they cruise through menopause with few or no symptoms. However, that leaves a huge 85 percent who experience some or all of the symptoms: hot flashes, night sweats, sleep disturbance, irregular or heavy menses, vaginal discomfort (itching, dryness, soreness, or pain), headaches, or loss of memory. And one of the prime symptoms, as discussed, is women's general disinterest in sex. And no wonder, with all of that going on!

Menopause can start anywhere from the mid-thirties up to age sixty, with the average age between forty-seven and fifty-two. It can also occur suddenly if a woman has had a hysterectomy—surgical removal of her womb, if it includes her ovaries—sending her into immediate menopause. Sudden menopause can also be precipitated by a shock to the body, either physical or emotional, such as a severe drop in weight or the death of a loved one. Essentially, menopause is activated when the ovaries no longer make estrogen and progesterone, two hormones needed for a woman's fertility, and a woman is generally referred to as officially being in menopause when her menstrual periods have ceased for one year. The time period immediately prior is known as perimenopause, meaning "around menopause." Perimenopause starts with changes in the menstrual cycle—often this will be months of skipped periods punctuated by periods of excessive bleeding—so it's the actual time before menopause is reached. The average length of perimenopause is said to be about four years but can last anywhere from a few months to ten years.

Many women in their thirties and forties experience symptoms without even being aware of it. These may include fatigue, mood swings, depression and anxiety, unaccustomed irritability, and generally not feeling like yourself. Unless the ovaries have been surgically removed, estrogen levels do not diminish overnight; it's a gradual process. That's why many women may not even detect that they are in perimenopause, but simply think they are going a bit mad!

The hormonal system is so delicate that Leslie Kenton, author of *Passage to Power: Natural Menopause Revolution,* likens it to a never-ending symphony; as one "instrument" (hormone) comes to the fore, others recede into the background, the body always balancing and changing. A woman's estrogen and progesterone levels can change from one hour to the next and depend greatly on her thoughts, feelings, and emotions, as well as external events in her environment.

Definitions

Perimenopause begins when hormonal changes in the body and menstrual cycle start to occur. It continues until a woman's final menstrual period.

Menopause is the final menstrual cycle of a woman's life and signals the end of fertility. It is confirmed after twelve months with no menstruation.

Postmenopause is the time period after menopause.

As Kenton explains, the word *hormone* comes from a Greek word, *hormao,* which means "I excite." And this, she continues, is exactly what hormones do. "They are messenger chemicals made in minute quantities in the brain or in special endocrine glands, such as the thyroid, adrenals, pancreas, and ovaries—sometimes even in fat cells—and then carried in the bloodstream to distant parts of the body where they control, activate, and direct the ever-changing system and organ functions, urges, and feelings that are *you.*"

Kenton goes on to say that each woman is biochemically and spiritually unique, noting that, "So central are hormonal events to how women think and feel that it would be no exaggeration to say the female endocrine system is an interface between body and spirit."* The hormones estrogen and progesterone work in close communication with the female body's control centers, the pituitary (the "master" gland, a tiny gland in the base of your brain), and the hypothalamus, known as the master "switchboard" because it's the part of the brain that controls the endocrine system. There are many hormones, but it's the "steroid" hormones, such as cortisol, progesterone, DHEA, testosterone, and estrogen, that are most closely associated with sex and reproduction for

---

*Leslie Kenton, *Passage to Power: Natural Menopause Revolution* (London: Random House, 1995), 59.

women. These steroid hormones are derived from cholesterol and have a big influence on the way we feel.

Hypothalamus

The hypothalamus is the control center. It balances and oversees biochemical and energetic changes throughout the body. The limbic system in which it sits is the most primitive part of the brain. It is the part that deals with the emotions and with our sense of smell, with our passions, and with all the unconscious interfaces that take place between mind and body. The actions of the limbic system lie beneath the level of the thinking mind. This is one of the reasons that the hypothalamus is often referred to as the "seat of the emotions." When excited the hypothalamus triggers desire—for food, for water, for adventure, for sex. Its actions can also be influenced by inhibitory thought patterns. If a woman is frightened about becoming pregnant, for instance, the fear itself—via the hypothalamus—can dampen sexual desire or even disrupt the menstrual cycle so she remains barren.

The hypothalamus even reacts to bodily changes that take place as a result of meditation. Its activities are also influenced by spiritual practices, which is a major reason why women who meditate regularly tend to develop greater emotional balance, as well as why repeated experiences of joy or stillness can dramatically improve various female complaints, such as PMS and hot flushes, in both menstruating and menopausal women.*

---

*Kenton, *Passage to Power*, 61.

Because the brain is involved, feedback from the endocrine system is altered, so any part of the body system—for example the digestive, nervous, or immune system—that is not working fully is going to affect every other part of the system. The response, in other words, will be holistic. As mentioned, biochemically all women are different.

However, there are factors that increase a woman's susceptibility to the more unpleasant ravages of menopause. This may simply be genetics, but more often it is lifestyle choices: nutrition and health, level of self-care, and stress. Studies have shown that chronic, long-term stress can cause menopause-like symptoms due to increased cortisol levels. In addition, the menopause process itself, with its myriad of symptoms and discomfort, can also cause stress for some women.

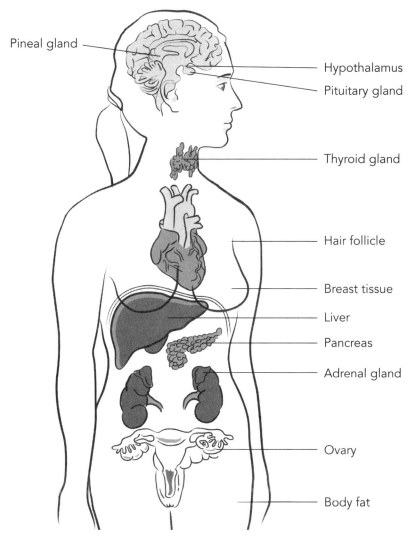

Fig. 2.1. Body sites capable of producing hormones

WHY THE BODY STARTS TO CHANGE

As mentioned, the hormonal system is complex, so we will provide a simple explanation here. Depending on factors of health, lifestyle, and genetics, sometime in a woman's thirties or forties her ovaries begin to slow their production of estrogen, which is the sexual and reproductive hormone. Estrogen controls a woman's monthly cycle. It enables a girl to develop into an adult woman, initiating the changes and growth of breasts as well as pubic and underarm hair, and heralds the beginning of menstruation. As estrogen controls the menstrual cycle, it is crucial to fertility. It also keeps cholesterol under control and helps protect bone health (as does progesterone). Estrogen is primarily produced in the ovaries, which produce the eggs. It's interesting to learn that the adrenal glands also produce some estrogen, as do our fat cells. Once created, estrogen is then transported to the body's tissues through our blood.

Lower Estrogen Levels

As menopause approaches, the ovaries begin to slow, causing lower levels of estrogen production. This results in symptoms such as irregular or absent periods, painful sex due to lack of vaginal lubrication, increase in urinary tract infections from thinning of the urethra, mood swings, headaches, difficulty concentrating, and fatigue.

Stress, Increased Anxiety, Sleep Difficulties, Fatigue

As estrogen levels begin to diminish, the reduced estrogen sends a bio-feedback signal to the brain, which then starts scrambling for more estrogen from other parts of the body, thus affecting other organs. Since the ovaries are not sending their usual feedback of estrogen to the kidneys or the adrenal and thyroid glands, the lower reptilian brain, the survival brain, responds to a perception that the body is under stress. Now it produces more stress hormones, which make the heart rate increase, which causes palpitations. In response, the higher brain starts releasing stress hormones, with the adrenals pumping cortisol.

This explains why women can feel nervous or have increased anxiety as menopause approaches, without any real explanation. "Like hot flashes, palpitations can range from mild to severe. They are rarely dangerous, though they can sometimes be very frightening. They are the result of the imbalance between the sympathetic and parasympathetic nervous systems, triggered by stress hormones, and are often related to fear and anxiety. If they persist, see your doctor."*

When the higher brain releases stress hormones and the adrenals start pumping cortisol, constant stress prevents the cortisol levels from returning to normal. This can result in too much cortisol continuing to circulate in the body, thus increasing anxiety. Or there can be too little cortisol if the adrenal glands become chronically fatigued.

Many a modern Western woman's condition is adrenal fatigue. Throughout all this the liver is working overtime. It has the capacity to transform the "anti-aging" hormone DHEA, produced by the adrenal glands, into any hormone the body needs. (The one exception is progesterone, which is a precursor to DHEA. That's why it is called the "mother hormone,'" which we will explain soon.) DHEA is a hormone that functions as a precursor to the male and female sex hormones, estrogen and testosterone, all needed to maintain vital healthy body function. DHEA production peaks in the mid-twenties, and the body's natural levels of sex hormones drop after that time. But when the body is producing a lot of stress hormone, it produces less DHEA, which obviously then lowers the sex response, due to the drop in sex hormones.

Stress Depletes Progesterone
All of this combined with the increased stress hormones affects the ability of the body to relax, unwind, and go to sleep at night. Therefore the menopausal woman is not getting restorative sleep, or she awakens

---

*Christiane Northrup, M.D., *The Wisdom of Menopause: Creating Physical and Emotional Health during the Change* (New York: Bantam Books, 2012), 143.

at 3 a.m., unable to return to sleep, and is then exhausted the next day. And so it continues in a vicious cycle. Women who fall prey to this cycle are at risk of spiraling in a downward direction. However, the body is actually designed to regulate itself, and often it will rebound if we give it a little help.

On the upside, many women have reported that the wee morning hours have become their most creative time if they get up and start writing or do some other creative activity. In traditional Chinese medicine (TCM), 3 to 5 a.m. is the "lung time." The lung is responsible for moving *qi* (energy) throughout the body, and helps with the immune function. The lung is also associated with the heart—grief, sadness, regret, or anything weighing heavily on the heart may emerge at this time. It's good to recognize and honor such feelings as they arise.

Too Much Estrogen

The reduction in progesterone in perimenopause and menopause can cause an estrogen dominance. Symptoms of estrogen dominance include headaches, anger and irritability, breast tenderness, hot flashes, weight gain, depression, mood swings, irregular cycles, heavy bleeding, painful periods, bloating, high blood pressure, and breast tumor formation, just to name a few. Many women are suffering difficult menopause due to this imbalance, possibly aggravated by lifestyle and environmental factors that are now pointing to an oversupply of estrogen in our bodies.

Use of chemicals and hormones in food production, which go into the food we consume, as well as contamination of the water we drink by prescription drugs, including estrogen from the Pill and HRT, can affect the delicate human endocrine system. Exacerbating the problem are common phenomena frequently occurring in most of our lives: overheated nonstick cookware leeches endocrine-disrupting chemicals into food. Off-gassing flame-retardants, anything from construction material to carpets, furniture, paint, and household goods, release similar types of chemicals into the environment. Heat causes chemical reactions in plastic water bottles and containers that also leech into food and water. All of these, including common household cleaners and personal care products, can potentially cause imbalances in the human body and are particularly disruptive for women.

The good news is that the body has an amazing capacity to heal and reverse symptoms when given the chance, and when supported in the right way by being mindful of eliminating these risk factors in your life and supporting your body to heal and return to balance.

Progesterone—It's Vitally Important

One powerful way to balance estrogen is with adequate amounts of progesterone. Progesterone has been around for 500 million years. It has been found in all vertebrates—fishes, reptiles, birds, and mammals, which include humans—and is essential for life. Researchers have found that many ailments and diseases can be remedied by adequate progesterone in the body.

As the ovaries stop ovulating, they stop producing progesterone. A cycle in which a woman is not ovulating can happen at any time in her life, but women often begin to skip ovulating by their mid-thirties. Estrogen can drop by about 35 percent when a woman enters menopause, but progesterone can plummet up to 95 percent or more. Because it affects how she feels, this loss can leave a woman feeling quite compromised, if not completely sideswiped by the more negative and troubling symptoms.

For women who suffer from the common complaints of depression, anxiety, hot flashes, weight gain, and so forth, progesterone could be a game changer. Progesterone has a soothing effect on the body and is a natural antidepressant, which makes it vitally important for women moving through menopause. It promotes good sleep and can sooth edginess, anxiety, and panic. It is an essential raw material for life and is a precursor hormone, meaning it has the ability to be turned into other hormones, such as testosterone and estrogen, among others.

Therefore, it is referred to as the "mother hormone." It protects against the negative effects of estrogen dominance, as described above. It can also bring surges of libido. We can see the effects of higher progesterone in a healthy woman in her third trimester of pregnancy; she is glowing, happy, and positive.

Progesterone is imperative for healthy bones and helps prevent osteoporosis. While estrogen prevents bone breakdown, it is progesterone that actually promotes bone building. It encourages fat burning instead of the tendency of estrogen to increase body fat, can help guard against breast cancer or cancer of the womb, and reduces blood clotting; thus it is an important factor in cardiac health for women.

Primarily made in the ovaries, progesterone is also made in the adrenal glands and can be converted into cortisol. Since stress fires off the fight-or-flight signal to the brain, it can cause excessive cortisol, which lowers progesterone levels. Large meals can also deplete progesterone levels, so smaller meals and avoiding eating too late at night will help you sleep better.

HORMONE REPLACEMENT THERAPY

Hormonal balancing is a very complex and individual issue. There are plenty of options ranging from traditional Hormone Replacement Therapy (HRT) to bioidentical hormones, and many natural herbal remedies and nutritional supplements, including those used by TCM (traditional Chinese medicine) and traditional herbal medicine. Many women have experienced great relief from perimenopausal, menopausal, postmenopausal, and indeed premenstrual symptoms using these supports. It is worth researching more about the natural ways to balance hormones if you're having trouble with symptoms, as each woman is unique.

Currently, the safety of over-the-counter hormone products (traditional HRT) is deeply questioned by some medical doctors who prefer to prescribe FDA-approved bioidentical hormones. This is largely due to the hazardous effects on women through the 1980s and '90s when HRT was composed of unopposed estrogen—that is, estrogen not partnered with progesterone or progestin, resulting in an increase in breast cancers and cardiac problems.

Bioidentical Hormones

Bioidentical hormones have been synthesized from plant sources and their molecular structure is identical to that of hormones in the human body. Doctors who are trained in the use of bioidentical hormones will test your hormone levels and may write a specific prescription for replacement of whatever hormone is deficient, such as progesterone, estrogen, DHEA, or testosterone. This can be made up by a compounding pharmacist that is a state-licensed pharmacist using FDA-approved bioidentical hormones.

The late John Lee, M.D., a pioneer in the research of bioidentical hormones, found that progesterone is so important as the precursor of all other hormones that the only thing women may need is to supplement with a high-quality bioidentical progesterone cream or tablets. Included in his protocol are specific nutritional supplements, regular gentle exercise, and good nutrition. Leslie Kenton has recorded his research in her book *Passage to Power.*

Dr. Northrup gives a very good analysis of bioidentical hormones and the importance of progesterone in *The Wisdom of Menopause.* See the back of this book for resources. It must be noted that a safe bioidentical alternative may be to supplement with a high-quality bioidentical progesterone cream produced by a good compounding pharmacist. Many women also report that wild yam cream works wonders to relieve their symptoms.

The biggest indicator of what is or isn't working is how you are feeling. If you are on progesterone and feel good, keep taking what you have been taking. If you do not, see your doctor. It's possible you may need another alternative, but in general, many women do seem to feel better on progesterone.

A Holistic Approach

Chinese medicine also offers a sound holistic approach to balancing the female system and has been used successfully for thousands of years. An experienced TCM practitioner can diagnose a woman's state of health and treat accordingly with acupuncture and effective herbal medicines. Others may prefer an Ayurvedic approach. As previously mentioned, every woman's body is unique and will respond differently to treatment, so it's wise to research and experiment. Ultimately intuition and a sense of well-being will reveal what works and feels best for your body.

Open the *Chi* Channels

In traditional Chinese medicine the kidneys are the source of our spirit (*shen*) and our life-force energy (*chi*). If they are compromised, the life-force energy stagnates and cannot flow to other areas of the body. Acupuncture opens the body's meridians and helps the energy channels to flow. Practices such as yoga, t'ai chi, and chi kung are also beneficial for moving stagnation.

Notice Your Feelings

Something that we and other women we know have noticed is that if you reflect on the split second *before* a hot flash, it is often associated with a thought or feeling that has arisen even before being conscious of it. Sometimes anger or fear or sadness—some kind of strong emotion—can trigger the sudden onset of a hot flash, which shows how closely associated our feelings are to our hormonal system. Note also what foods you have eaten prior to having these sudden rises of heat in your body and you might find that your body is telling you what exacerbates them and what might appease them.

Hot Flashes and the Liver

Cleansing the liver is very helpful for menopause.

One woman shares her experience with liver detox:

I thought I was going crazy. My emotions were all over the place. I went from loving mother to screaming banshee. I was desperate and ended up at a naturopath seeking any kind of help. She immediately put me onto a liver detox and herbs, and I have never looked back. Within a short period of time, all my symptoms, including hot flashes, reduced substantially. I felt like my old self again.

THE RESTORATIVE POWER OF LOVEMAKING

If the negative effects of stress and lifestyle have a lot to do with how a woman moves through menopause, any change that balances the whole system, such as meditation, yoga, t'ai chi, or a more relaxed style of lovemaking, holds an essential key for contemporary women. Making love in relaxation soothes and calms the nervous system of the perimenopausal and menopausal woman in a beautiful and natural way. One of the keys to creating this relaxed state in lovemaking may be familiar to mindfulness practitioners—simply bringing awareness to the present. When one is fully present to the immediate moment, all thoughts of past and future become peripheral or vanish. This has been the ultimate aim of all meditation practice: being in the present moment. By this definition, making love moment by moment can itself be a meditation.

Changing the way we make love challenges our past ideas of conventional sex and leads us into a world of wonder where deep healing and restoration of the body and spirit is possible. If we keep relaxation as a staple, a constant, in our approach to making love, then we start to open our minds and hearts to a more inner experience of sex. Because a woman's ability to relax has a vast influence on her hormonal balance, it goes without saying that making love in a relaxed manner can indeed help to balance a woman's overall health.

Conscious, slow sex and making love in relaxation generate a restorative effect in the parasympathetic nervous system, the rest-and-digest response, which is part of the greater autonomic nervous system responsible for involuntary functions in the body. Once the body is restored to balance it can usually make enough DHEA, the youth-rejuvenating hormone, on its own. Studies show that after one month of using the HeartMath system,* which is basically breathing in and out of your heart center with positive thoughts, DHEA levels increase dramatically and levels of cortisol reduce significantly. This has a positive effect on the whole functioning of the body.

Therefore directing awareness and intention to the breasts during lovemaking, as we will expand on in chapter 7, naturally activates and engages the heart, which then involves the whole body. By activating the healing power of the parasympathetic nervous system, one can extrapolate that it may automatically increase DHEA levels, therefore balancing and healing the whole endocrine system. This naturally restores harmony in the body's systems, and we have repeatedly found, both in our own experiences and those reported by others, that making love in awareness and relaxation also positively balances a woman's fluctuating emotional states, and therefore her hormones.

Hopefully you now understand the importance of hormones, especially for women who suffer in any way or have suffered during the menstrual years. The balance of estrogen and progesterone in particular can have a major life impact. For the woman who is feeling great, there's no need to change anything. But for the woman who's not, it's important to remember the holistic approach: preventive lifestyle and nutritional choices, stress, emotional health, the state of relation-

---

*HeartMath is a system of techniques designed to transform stress and develop the heart's intelligence.

ships, and the surrounding environment and environmental toxins all have an influence. Most important, every woman should do more of what makes her happy! Whatever supports the amazing hormones and allows a woman to ride the wave of menopause with ease will be of tremendous benefit.

◻ Recommended Restorative Yoga Positions

Yoga offers much for a woman of any age to help balance the endocrine system. The following *asanas,* or poses, are particularly good for replenishment and for pacifying the adrenal glands. All the yoga poses in this book can be used as a gentle sequence or as stand-alone postures.

Wide-Legged Supported Child Pose
(*Balasana*)

Forward bend is very soothing for the adrenal glands and calms all systems of the body. Turn your head to each side to balance out the neck. It's worth investing in a bolster to support your menopause journey (can be bought from any yoga supply outlet). Try adapting this with a chair if you have trouble with knees or hips.

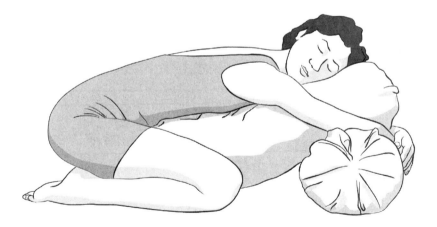

Fig. 2.2. Wide-Legged Supported Child Pose

Reclining Supported Simple Cross-Legged Pose
(*Supta Sukhasana*)

This pose promotes a calm mind and is soothing for the whole system. It creates spaciousness in the belly and opens the heart and chest. It also increases blood supply to the pelvis, bathing and bringing nourishment to the reproductive organs.

Note: *Not to be done while menstruating.* It can help with mood swings and can relieve menstrual cramping when done *only* around the time of ovulation.

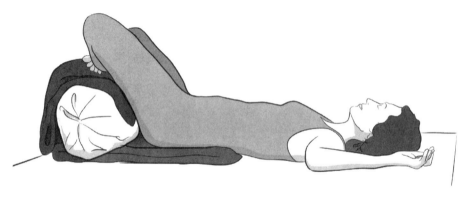

Fig. 2.3. Reclining Supported
Simple Cross-Legged Pose

Corpse Pose
(*Savasana*)

This pose helps relieve anxiety, nervous tension, and hot flashes, and is deeply replenishing. Placing your hands on your lower belly, breathe slowly into your abdomen three times, feeling your lower abdomen lifting and lowering your hands with the rise and fall of your breath. Then place your hands over your ribs at each side of your chest. Practice upper-body or thoracic breathing slowly three times, feeling your hands moving in and out with each breath. Then relax completely.

When you have practiced this a few times, you may find there is no need to place your hands on your body. Simply let them lie relaxed at your sides as you start with the breathing each time. And then proceed with relaxation. This will help bring equilibrium to your nervous system and calm you. Stay in this pose for at least five minutes.

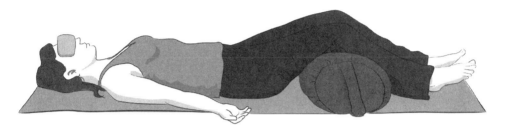

Fig. 2.4. Corpse Pose

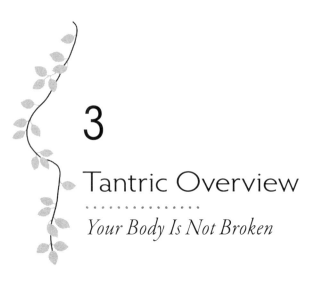

3

Tantric Overview

Your Body Is Not Broken

AS EACH WOMAN'S JOURNEY THROUGH menopause is individual, it is impossible to make all-embracing statements about it because so many threads weave into the fabric of personal experience, including culture, genetics, lifestyle, attitude, and life story. At the same time women share in common many highly significant aspects of menopause. This means that a lot of information can be passed on to make the passage easier and empower women, whether they are in a partnership or on their own. Being offered an alternative perspective on female sexuality establishes an increased level of self-understanding and self-trust. So as unique as women's experience may be, the journey is also a universal one, and menopause is inevitable for all women who live beyond their childbearing years.

Even so, as natural an unfolding as this process is, if not encouraged otherwise, women can tend to have tremendous despondency with regard to aging, sex, and menopause. Many women feel themselves to be deficient or lacking in something, and frequently experience a very low sense of self-worth, as if they are no longer "seen." Many women report that they actually feel sexually "broken." Unfortunately much of this despondency is simply due to not having access to important information about male and female sexual energies, their differences, and the way they complement each other at a fundamental level—a level that supports a woman's body and her innate sexual design.

Those women who transit menopause with great ease may nonetheless yearn for more depth and connection in their sexual relationships. Some women enjoy a new freedom in their sexual aliveness, liberated from monthly bleeding cycles, yet seem to have trouble finding men who can meet them on a deeper level in this newfound awakening. Whatever category a woman falls into, there is a drive in the modern woman to have more and to be more. Although there is nothing wrong with such longings per se, actively striving for them can ultimately divert a woman from her essential nature, making it more likely that she feels disoriented. The answer may lie in a new level of inner anchoring and inner perception that lies deep within her.

TRUST YOUR OWN BODY

In the coming chapters we endeavor to explain and share with you the possibility of how your attitude to your body, and your understanding of female sexuality, can transform you and awaken what is available to you at this inherently exciting and rich time of your life. We explore the power that this time of change represents for a woman, and what's possible when she turns her awareness inward to her own inner life. Women who participate in our retreats often give us feedback after a few days, saying, "I knew this information all along but I did not trust it," as if the notion were something already hidden within their bodies, within their very genetics.

What occludes this knowing and disturbs the trust in our bodies? Basically it's our sexual conditioning, as explained previously, as well as our general lack of body awareness as humans. We are more in our minds and in mechanical thinking mode than in our bodies and feeling, sensing mode. The way we have made love for centuries has been without attention to the intrinsic energetic qualities of male and female polarities, and with little thought of the holistic and healing potential of sex, beyond its reproduction function. Basically we have lost connection to, and faith in, our own bodies, lost the capacity to listen, follow, and flow with its many impulses, messages, and signals.

INTRODUCING TANTRA

Tantra has become increasingly popular in recent years. However, there are different levels, interpretations, and associations that can potentially cause confusion. The word itself derives from India's ancient Sanskrit language and means "expansion of energy, expansion of consciousness, web of consciousness." For us, Tantra is essentially this: the ancient art of awareness (mindfulness) applied to the self and to the body in daily life as well as in sex, which ideally is part of daily life. In Tantra sex is not practiced for its own sake, as indulgence or entertainment, but as an instrument for going *beyond* sex, for reaching health, balance, improved couple relationships, self-control, and eventually superior states of consciousness. The tantric practice of sexual reabsorption allows for the conversion and elevation of the huge sexual potential, producing rapid and beneficial transformation of the human being. And this exploration begins with accessing the innate "magnetic" intelligence anchored in our hearts and genitals.

Awareness directed into the body creates expansion rather than contraction, and requires being conscious moment by moment rather than mechanically repeating patterns. The miracle of awareness (or mindfulness) is that it has the power to transform life, dramatically improve its quality, and increase self-love and joy. Tantric awareness amplifies sensuality and can be brought into play at any time of the day (or night!), either with a partner or independent of a partner. And this moment-to-moment awareness is especially powerful when incorporated into lovemaking.

Equal and Opposite Poles
The essence of tantric knowledge is that each individual forms a complete "magnetic unit." The body carries two equal and opposite energy

poles: one in the heart/chest area, and one in the genital area. One pole is male, which is inherently dynamic, or "positive," and has the power to raise energy and awaken vitality. It's important to note that the word "dynamic" in this context does not mean active or refer to activity. Dynamic means there is an inherent capacity to flow that occurs without actively doing anything; it arises of its own accord and comes into play when an environment conducive to its response is created. At times this may happen spontaneously, but it is possible through awareness to consciously create the situation.

The corresponding female pole is inherently receptive, or "negative," with the power to absorb, to take in, to receive. Here again it's important to note that "receptive" in this context does not mean passive or unengaged. It means to be fully present, yet nondoing. And these two powers—dynamic and receptive—are equal forces, while at the same time they are opposite forces that complement each other and work in unison as a single unit, as two parts of one whole.

In the last few decades the truth that each individual carries both male and female chromosomes has been scientifically established. However, Tantra's understanding of these complementary aspects dates back more than ten thousand years.

Rod of Magnetism

The presence of these two equal and opposite internal forces forms a very important biomagnetism that gives rise to a kind of inner magnet. This "rod of magnetism" enables energy and vitality to circulate and stream throughout the body. Effectively, we are all able to circulate sexual/life/chi energy within ourselves, and independent of a partner. Internally this self-sustaining magnetic energy circulates through the body and connects the positive and negative poles. Tuning in to this fine, delicate, and subtle level of inner reality enables every individual to self-nourish and replenish, independent of sex. Basically we are designed in an auto-ecstatic way, meaning each individual has the capacity to circulate blissful energies within, which ironically is considered the highest or most evolved form of sex. It is so helpful for women who are transiting menopause with or without partners to understand their bodies as a resource that can bring a lot of joy and happiness.

Engaging with self in this auto-ecstatic way can lead to heightened states in which an expansion of energy is experienced through the magnetic field that surrounds the body. When the awareness expands beyond the physical body, orgasmic or blissful or ecstatic states can occur in which peace and harmony prevail, where time dissolves in pure presence, as if embraced by the arms of the universe. Such experiences are highly revitalizing, energizing, uplifting, and unforgettable. Whether alone or with a partner, we melt and merge with our own bodies.

Even for those with a partner, ultimately the vitality is circulating within each individual, independent of the other person. This view certainly creates more independence, especially for someone who may be thinking it's about having a significant other.

Reader Suzanna shares her awakening:

A few years back I had lost all interest in sex. I felt completely broken as a woman. Yet deep down inside, there was a kind, soft voice telling me I was not broken and there was nothing wrong with me, I just needed to find the key to unlocking my inner fire. Then life as I knew it began to implode as my marriage came apart at the seams. To cope with the stress I started to meditate, which is to say I sat still in silence for about fifteen minutes a day listening for that internal kind, soft, guiding voice. During a meditation one night I entered a state of orgasmic bliss that lasted what seemed like an impossibly long time. It was a total game-changer. I suddenly understood that there was something really powerful I could tap into inside, and that sexual pleasure was more about my own inner vitality than about the activities we do together with our bodies. I found your book, Tantric Orgasm for Women,* shortly after my initial awakening and it was a beacon of light on my lonely journey. The information*

---

*Diana Richardson, *Tantric Orgasm for Women* (Rochester, Vt.: Destiny Books, 2004).

you presented and the way you presented it really spoke to me and helped me move through some limiting beliefs surrounding my sexual potential. I finally felt someone was explaining the unfulfilled sexual experience I'd had all my adult life.

Poles Reversed in Male and Female Bodies

One of the magnetic poles is in the chest/heart area and the other pole is in the genitals. The dynamic "plus" pole is the life-giving, energy-raising positive pole from which aliveness flows to the equal and opposite receptive "minus" pole, at least in its initial stages. It must be noted here that *plus* and *minus* are figurative terms and do not imply that one is more or better than the other. In women it is obvious that the breasts are the positive energy-raising or life-giving/sustaining pole. In the male body it's equally obvious that the life-giving pole is in the penis/testicles. Conversely, a man's receptive pole is in the heart/chest area, and a woman's receptive pole is the vagina.

Women's Energy-Raising Pole

Energy and vitality is "raised" from a plus pole, and not from a minus pole. However, in the usual approach to sex, a woman's vagina, and especially the clitoris, is conventionally considered to be the center of female sexuality. Yes, it's true in the sense that the clitoris is sensitive and creates intensity and excitement, but this is not the way a woman's body opens deeply, not where her deeper, more subtle sexual energy is raised, and not how her body awakens according to a deeper magnetic design. This completely contradicts current views about the clitoris, and only firsthand experience will lead you to question this belief.

The deeper opening of a woman's body happens via the breasts and nipples, and then, *given the time,* will be felt as a vibrational resonance or response that opens the vagina and makes the tissues receptive. Engaging a woman's body on this energetic level brings her to a true willingness, where she no longer submits to sex but participates fully.

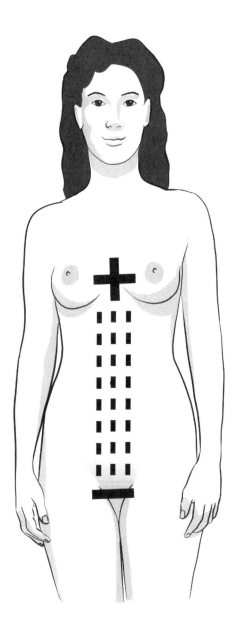

Fig. 3.1. Dynamic and receptive poles at breasts and vagina
respectively, illustrating the magnetic rod

Sexual Temperature

It's very important to understand that because the awakening happens in the upper body, time is naturally required for a melting into the breasts and the flow and spreading of vitality to the lower body. When this occurs, there is a deep yes to receiving; a woman longs to have the man enter her, to take him inside her. Because of the lack of time and understanding in conventional sex, with the focus on the clitoris, a woman's body seldom opens to its full potential, and thus begins the process of a gradual physical closing down. A woman's loss of interest (after the sexual intensity of the honeymoon phase) is often mistakenly interpreted as frigidity, or being blocked in some way, physically or psychologically. The woman, too, thinks there is something really wrong with her because she can't open up and be ready for sex instantly.

When a woman's body is honored as it is designed by nature—understanding that her body opens differently from a man's and her sexual temperature rises much more slowly than his—then the woman is totally and absolutely happy to make love, her interest returns, and she begins to shine with love. Countless times we have witnessed this during our couples' retreats. From a starting point of feeling disconnected from a partner, and sometimes not having made love for years, within three days of exploring new sexual territory using new guidelines, there is a huge shift from disinterest to being fully engaged and enthusiastic. What this reveals is that it is not sex per se that is the problem, it's more about how we usually go about having sex.

Figure 3.2 on page 40 shows how the inner magnets of man and woman correspond and fit together because opposite poles are meeting: man's positive lower body pole meets woman's positive upper body pole. So for example, when man and woman stand opposite each other, effectively they are like two magnets meeting at opposite ends, and the magnets exert a force on each other. So additionally, beyond the individual inner magnetic set up, there is the potential for a circular path and flow and exchange of energy between male and female

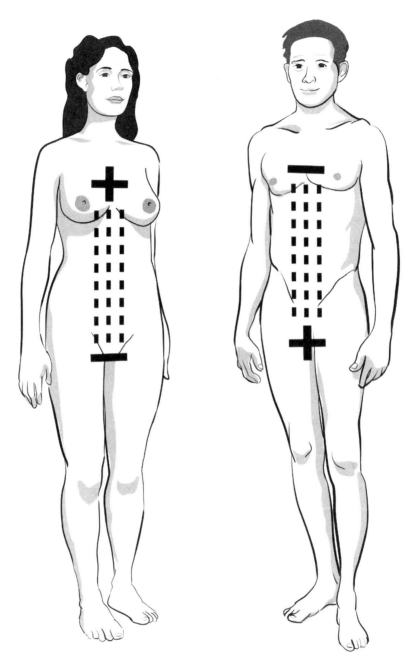

Fig. 3.2. Female and male bodies showing
opposite polarities and the rods of magnetism

bodies, as well as an expansion of the magnetic field surrounding the bodies.

While the figure shows the correspondence of male and female bodies, it is the accessing of inner aliveness as an individual that has priority, and this means that subtle flows and exchanges of energy can also be experienced between female-female bodies and male-male bodies.

Female Body in Its Totality Is Receptive

It helps to understand that as women, even though inwardly we contain both male/dynamic and female/receptive forces, outwardly on a global body energy level we are female, receptive, and absorbing. And the same is true for men. Inwardly both forces are present, yet, outwardly a man's body energy has a dynamic, flowing, moving quality.

Beginning to understand the receptive powers of her own unique composition and responding to the dynamic force of male flowing toward her or within her or through her opens new doors for a woman. And as already mentioned, it's vital to understand that receptivity is not something to be done and it's not passive and inert; receiving is the intrinsic capacity to take in and absorb, to become a passage. And receptivity is a very powerful force.

It's All Within You

The discovery of the subtle level of magnetic aliveness lying within holds a vital key to the menopausal woman's journey. Once a woman understands her inner design and then actually experiences it within her own self (alone or with another), the menopausal woman, and in fact every woman, whatever age she is, can become liberated on an inner level, which then affects how she moves into the world.

For women who are experiencing menopause at present, what it means is this: there is nowhere you need to go to seek what you are yearning for, for it is already here, anchored right in your very own body. For many years in our Making Love Retreats, over and over we have seen women break down in tears from the relief at hearing this foundational interpretation of Tantra. They realize that they simply are not broken or deficient, and that their disinterest in sex is not to do with their bodies—they are not congested or uptight. They are just different! The way the female body opens and readies itself for sex is very, very different from the way the male body opens. And there is certainly a style of sex that is well suited to woman's body energy and her hormonal changes; however, it is different from the accepted style of conventional or traditional sex.

A retreat participant shares her experiences:

I am an acupuncturist and specialize in menopause. After I experienced several years of postmenopausal vaginal dryness and low sex drive, my husband and I decided to attend the Making Love retreat. I had low expectations that anything would change . . . to me it seemed like my vagina was damaged beyond repair. I was extremely pleasantly surprised that I quickly opened like a flower when I understood that the female body requires a longer time to warm up than a male body, and that for women the breasts are the energy-awakening pole in the body. As a result, my vaginal tissues have regenerated and I am eager for intimacy. I can feel energy pulsing throughout my body and opening my heart. Making love has become so yummy and revitalizing!!!!! I am so surprised at how quickly this has happened!!!!

Impact of Sexual Conditioning

Sex as we know it has been informed and impacted by our sexual conditioning. The imprints of all the misunderstandings about sex that we inherit from our society on an unconscious level start from our earliest years. These sexual patterns and imprints have distracted all of us from our true natures. Of course logically we know that women's bodies and men's bodies are different, but it's the actual way sexual energy arises in the female body, and how that life force moves through and prepares our bodies, that holds the key.

Invert Attention

It is common in our society to be immensely busy directing our energy outward, away from our center. We are tremendously outwardly focused on plans, on getting ahead, on getting results, on setting up and reaching our goals. Similarly, the style in which we make love conventionally goes in this direction too. We are more focused on the other than on ourselves, more outside of our bodies than inside of our bodies. And in sex, we are often more focused on a climax, which usually marks the end of sex, than being present and letting things be and unfold.

In place of the habitual outward movement of attention and energy, we make suggestions throughout this book to replace it with the opposite, with an inversion of your attention to inside the body as an anchor point for your awareness. Internally this attitude and level of mindfulness can indefinitely and substantially nourish you at this important time of your life and as you advance into your later years. With the understanding that there is nowhere you need to go to seek what you are yearning for, a new sense of self-worth can start to fill you up and flow through your body. Tuning in to the subtle aliveness, ever present within you, is like having a light suddenly switched to the "on" position. We see women (within a couple of days) start to blossom like the delicate, yet strong and beautiful, flowers they truly are. Metaphorically speaking, they appear to grow quite rapidly from seedling to flower in grace and confidence.

YOUR BODY IS PERFECT AS IT IS

If you have felt, or feel, as if you are broken, that your body doesn't work anymore, that it doesn't work as well as it used to when you had raging hormones in your younger years, we are here to reassure you quite loudly that it does! And it works perfectly and beautifully, just differently. Through the explanation we give, you will come to know that clearly. You're not broken. You are simply going through a natural change, a natural phase of womanhood, and potentially one of the most powerful times of your life. There's just less drive in a woman's body to reproduce now that the hormones are not running around frantically looking to mate.

Women interpret that as being deficient. It's simply hormones changing the biological response, but there is a far greater power that can come with this period of life. A quieter and more inward silence is available now, and there's a different type of power in that. Ease and grace replace headiness and the intoxicating flood of revved-up reproductive hormones. The natural potential within the body and heart are alive right now. It is simply a matter of shifting your perspective to a more inner experiencing. Nature's arrangement of our hormones to create life is now moved to a level that allows our bodies to give birth to another kind of life, a life more of our choosing, of our own calling.

Women's problems during menopause and difficulties with having sex are seen as pathology in this modern age. We want to remove it from the pathological arena and raise it into the realm of health and well-being. And that requires a shift in attention, to look to what is innately healthy and alive in the body, instead of what "appears" wrong. This creates space for a shift in the psyche, and the inherent health of the body will follow.

An Energy Body, First and Foremost

What gives our bodies life is the life force, or chi. This is the energy body, albeit invisible. When we can reroute our attention inward, anchor and reference ourselves from inside rather than seeing ourselves from the outside (how we look, what we do for a living, whether we have a mate or not), there is new ground available to us as women. When our minds live only in the realm of the physical and the external, we forget the energetic reality of the body and its innate and holy potential, its capacity and intrinsic thrust to come into balance and wholeness. When the appropriate environment is created for the body to open at a deeper level, no matter what age, open it will.

◖ *Resting in Consciousness*

The aligned position for resting in consciousness is perhaps the most delightful and beneficial practice an individual can do (if you have a partner or not) on a regular or even daily basis. It is highly recommended because the awareness is turned inward and brings you and your body into focus. The practice needs a minimum of twenty to thirty minutes and is as simple as this:

Lie down, close your eyes, and bring your awareness within your body. It's important to lie with the spine, head, and neck in a straight line. You may need a flat pillow to support your head, but be sure that your head is not tilted upward. Alignment is crucial as it contributes tremendously to the level of your presence.

Place a pillow beneath the knees to support them, so they are slightly softened and curved, which will greatly enhance your capacity to enter into the body and relax.

If possible, turn your feet slightly inward rather than letting them fall outward in a V-shape; this also helps to connect to the lower body, which is so often out of our awareness.

Place your hands on your belly as shown in figure 3.3 on page 46, or you can put them on your groin area, or wrap them around the sides of your thighs.

When you are comfortable, turn your attention from outside to inside, leaving behind the thoughts of the day. Sweep through your whole body with the awareness, softening and relaxing any tension that you notice.

It can help to contract and tighten the body at first, exaggerating the tension and releasing it. Do this several times, contracting and relaxing. Sense the upper half of the body and then the lower half of the body, and unite them by holding your attention in the area above the navel, the solar plexus.

Slowly sink into the sensations of the body, looking inward and downward with your inner eye. Spread your attention evenly throughout your entire body, always keeping the head and neck in one line. Breathe deeply and slowly into the belly, and just "be." Give value to any subtle feelings of aliveness in your body, and don't look for great things!

This very specific body position will help you to sink inward and, after some time, enable your consciousness to move beyond the body's physical boundaries. When a union with the subtle energies in the body is achieved, time melts away, we become fully present to the moment, and inner contentment and fulfillment arise. We feel filled up from within, and fully refreshed and energized. (And we don't regret it so much if there's an empty space in the bed next to us!)

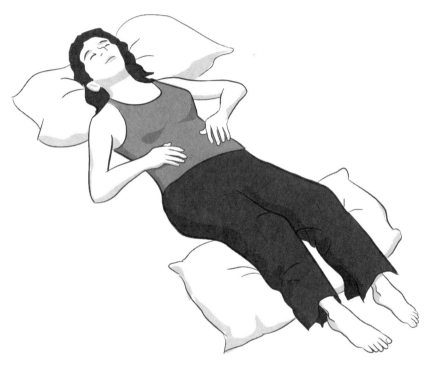

Fig. 3.3. Aligned body position for resting in consciousness

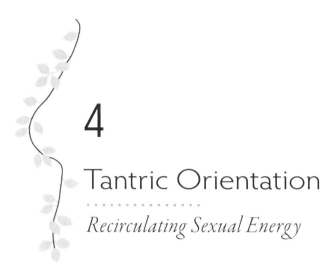

4

Tantric Orientation

Recirculating Sexual Energy

IN CONVENTIONAL SEX, stimulation of the genitals causes the usual orgasm or ejaculation and a release of energy downward. Commonly this stimulation is caused through high sensation, rising heat, and rapid movement. It is often fast and hot. Once there is a peak and discharge, this usually signals the end of the sex act. Any concept that sex can last for longer than twenty minutes or even forty minutes is often considered to be in the realm of exaggeration. The possibility that sex can go beyond this and not involve a peak is almost inconceivable.

THE SOURCE OF SEXUAL ENERGY

In conventional sex the mind and the imagination function as the fuel of sexual excitement. However, the real source of sexual energy resides in the pituitary and pineal glands, in the brain. These are considered to be the master glands of the body. They are like the control center for the entire endocrine system—the hormonal system of the body. The master glands secrete hormones that flow through the body in different levels, which allows blood to also flood the genital and pelvic area, causing arousal and preparing us for sexual exchange and pleasure.

Reproductive Phase

This initial phase of having sex when the sexual energy cycle begins in the brain, travels to the genitals, and then leaves the body in the downward release of orgasm is called the "reproductive phase" of sex (fig. 4.1). The biology of human reproduction is a miracle of life, a wonder to behold, and allows our species to survive generation to generation. That this sperm from a man's ejaculation can fertilize this egg within a woman's womb, begin the spark of conception, and gestate inside a woman's body to become another human being is truly a miracle. However, it requires a downward release of energy/semen for the wonder to complete itself. This is usually as far as general awareness goes with sex, but we are, in fact, living only one-half of our sexual potential.

Spiritual and Generative Phase

Human sexual design, via the inner rod of magnetism (see fig. 3.2 on page 40), grants us the possibility to transcend the reproductive function of sex and thereby move to higher elevated states. This is where tantric teachings have much to offer. And this is certainly some good news for a woman and her partner as she moves beyond her reproductive years, because this potential is as mysterious and revolutionary as reproduction itself, and it comes into being through changing the way we make love.

As humans we have been given the gift of conscious awareness and the cognitive ability to observe, think, and act beyond our instinctive reproductive responses. Animals have sex by coming into heat, through the production of hormones. Other than humans (and dolphins apparently), animals do not copulate for any reason but reproduction.

Human Choice, the Turning Point

As humans we have been given the opportunity to engage in the sex act at any time, whether we make babies or not. Of course the sharing of love, pleasure, and sensuality is the incentive. To have been given the opportunity to experience the heightened pleasure, sensitivity, deep bonding, and love that is possible during sex is the gift of living

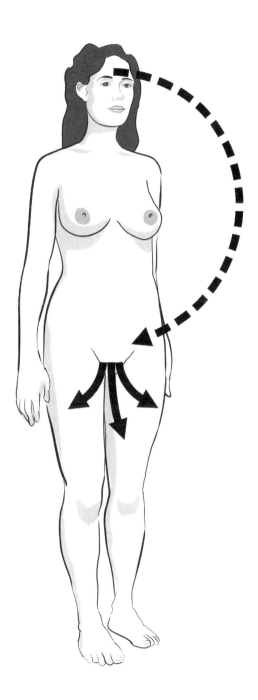

Fig. 4.1. Biological or reproductive phase of sexual energy—
downward and outward

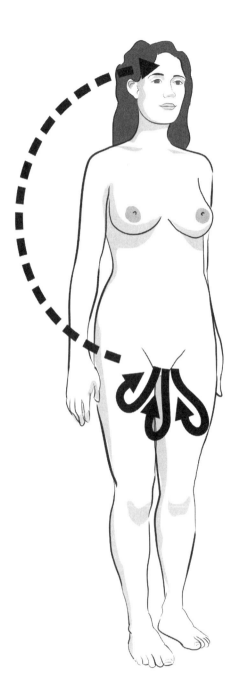

Fig. 4.2. Generative or spiritual phase of sexual energy—
inward and upward

in a human body. Because of our suppression and repression of the body and pleasure, the shame and guilt that often goes along with sex, opening to pleasure in and of itself can be a healing and life-giving, liberating experience. But in the end, if pleasure per se is the only goal, once reproduction is out of the picture, even that will leave us feeling empty.

Creative Energy Not Dispersed

When we allow for the circulation of sexual energy through not discharging it, the vitality returns to its source in the brain. This is called the spiritual or generative phase of sexual energy (fig. 4.2). So the creative energy is not escaping or dispersing from the body, which is what happens in orgasm and ejaculation, where the energy is lost through downward and outward movement. Discovering how to contain the energy (not to build energy to a peak) enables an upward circulation of vitality to its ultimate source in the brain, and this nourishes the master glands (see fig. 4.3 on page 52). This "backflow," or return flow to the brain, energizes the whole system and has a positive impact on health, the immune system, clarity, and creativity, and increases the sense of well-being. People report new insights into the self, new ways of looking at life, inspirations for projects, and a general widening of horizons, both inside and outside the bedroom.

So in a simple, natural, and organic way, through containing sexual energy a woman can start to reach her deeper, wiser nature and access her creativity. Her love expands in a way that may never have been experienced previously. She may even feel touched by the Divine. And such fulfilling experiences can finally give a woman true confidence in herself, in her body, and in her own love.

BENEFITS OF CONTAINMENT

For the woman seeking answers in her mid- to later life, tapping the higher potential of sex can help her gain access to territories she

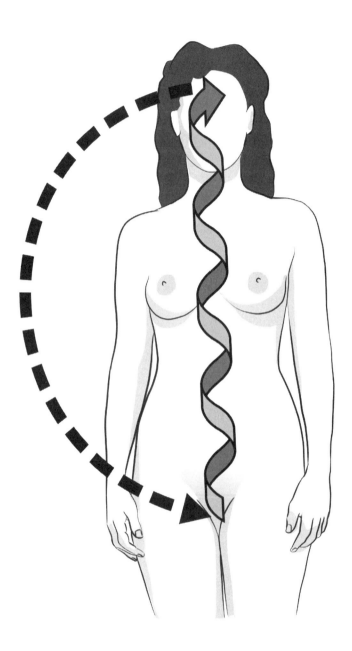

Fig. 4.3. Complete sexual energy circle
with redirected energy spiraling through energy centers
to reach the brain

intuitively yearns for. The key is, however, in harnessing and containing that vital energy that usually gets released downward. More concretely, it means breaking the habit and pattern of always going for a peak orgasm. Instead, in Tantra we create a relaxed lovemaking environment that encourages this vitality to be reabsorbed, thus bathing the entire body, genitals, endocrine system, brain, and every cell with the release of soothing chemicals (hormones) that actually regenerate both partners. That is why this aspect is called the "generative phase" of sex. Instead of building and releasing energy in an orgasm, the energy is retained and naturally circulates upward through the body with profound regenerating and healing effects.

Containment is created not by suppression of the sex energy, but through the simple (yet powerful) act of awareness and remaining relaxed during sex—that is, not working toward peak orgasms using tension and pressure. This enables the aliveness to expand through the body, which is designed for this occurrence. The sexual energy rises all by itself, provided it is contained through awareness and relaxation. When it is contained, this vitality stays inside you and the body does something else with it—it starts to rise naturally because you are not pushing the vitality downward and outward, as in regular orgasm.

This generative phase is also sometimes called the "spiritual phase" of sex because it has the power to initiate profound transformation; we begin a process of evolution and start to grow as individuals. This relaxation in the sex center is what transforms a woman from a submissive female to an empowered woman who knows her own value and the power of her receptive energy. In the same way, it transforms a restless man into a loving, centered man who is master of his dynamic energy.

Sex without Excitement?

The question naturally arises: How is it possible to engage sexually and stay relaxed? It's true that stimulation and tension create sensation and pleasure, but this is intensity, not expansion. And it is over so quickly, setting up a situation of never feeling satiated, caught in a cycle of desire and discharge, without deeper fulfillment. Those with a greater sex drive are left hungering for more, wanting the same thing again and again. The circle of sexual energy never completes itself and the body never gets a chance to benefit from being bathed by love and soothing chemicals. Moreover, sex is usually over far too quickly for a woman's body to have warmed up fully. This is due to the high tendency for premature ejaculation. She may often be left high and dry, looking at the ceiling while he has fallen fast asleep, wondering how much longer she can continue to do this. As exciting as it might be, the rewards leave little to inspire her. Invariably sex is over when the man ejaculates, which is often long before the woman is even close to orgasm. This is primarily because the global average from time of entry to male ejaculation is said to be about two and a half minutes. Sometimes a premature ejaculation is a relief for a woman, especially if she has given up hope of ever having anything different.

Basically it can be said that we humans are caught up in a peak-and-discharge style of sex: building excitement through stimulation, using tension and contraction to reach a peak of intensity, and then discharging the energy downward with millions of sperm per ejaculation. Nature gave us this for reproduction but not necessarily for everyday use. For a man, a tremendous amount of energy, spiritual and physical, is required to manufacture and replace the lost sperm.

Containing or Retaining Energy

Since we are not always looking to reproduce, we don't need to have reproductive-style sex every time. This realization is life changing. Instead of discharging, we can retain the vitality and start taking sex in a more easy and relaxed way, more conscious of what we do and how we do it. It's a level of awareness that naturally makes us more sensitive and draws us into the present moment. We can experiment with not pushing our bodies in a certain direction (the peak), but instead keeping things "cool" and avoiding raising the sexual temperature so that ejaculation is kept at bay. Certainly, in the beginning of this exploration, this coolness can be used to extend the lovemaking because ejaculation is likely to happen from time to time.

Interestingly, analysis of sperm has revealed that it contains micro amounts of gold, so essentially semen can be considered liquid gold! Gold is something to be preserved and cared for, not dispersed and discarded. On the contrary, it is extremely healthy and invigorating to refrain from habitual discharge of sexual fluids and instead contain the energy, for both women and men. As mentioned, the body is designed to recycle that sexual vitality and put it to other good uses. Even though women do not have sperm to replace, they also lose energy through orgasm due to the effort and tension involved in getting to the peak. It's a buildup and a release, and the vitality is discharged downward.

Sometimes a woman will have an orgasm without working for it at all; it happens by itself through relaxation. In this case there is usually no downward loss of energy. The experience is more likely to be a spreading and expansion inside the body.

Most women seldom have sufficient space and clock time for adequate body warming. A woman's sexual temperature rises more slowly than a man's, so her need or wish or longing to have "more time" before receiving the man into her is not because she is somehow iced over or has problems, but because of the intrinsic body magnetism and ways we are different from mens, as explained in chapter 3.

Pattern of Pleasing Men

Once real pleasure and loving connection is no longer possible for a woman, she may well resort to pleasing. All over the world women are strongly conditioned to please men, to keep them happy, even doing things that they know are not so loving to their own bodies. As already touched on, a woman can find herself in a double bind, caught between losing the relationship if she does not agree to sex and having sex purely to please him and maintain the status quo. Neither is a particularly viable option. No longer can she open her heart to her man, even though it may be her dearest wish to do so. No longer can she reveal her tender nature to herself, or to him.

This dampening of woman's essence gives rise to a tremendous sadness and a burning need or longing for more conscious love. It's as if the love that can't be expressed turns in on itself and becomes an ache inside her. Or she simply goes along in a kind of numb state, not really aware of feeling anything at all. This situation can also give rise to a powerful rage that can leak unhealthily into the relationship, leaving a man wondering what he has done wrong.

Questioning Convention

Both women and men frequently intuit that there must be more to sex; however, they don't trust themselves enough to experiment with something new and unknown, choosing instead to follow the imprinting, patterns, and expectations of conventional sex—a style of sex that is hot and intense, involving as much excitement as possible with lots of friction movements of penis inside vagina, all with the intention (goal) of producing a climax, which is inevitably followed by a discharge.

Until a woman begins to question this conventional pattern of sex, ignoring what she knows in her bones to be in true alignment with her body and being, couples can be stuck in a very difficult place. This is when the quest begins, whether a woman is twenty-six or fifty-six. When this voice rises from within, she must follow its tune. She knows there must be another way; she just doesn't know what or how.

A man, too, can be left confused and despondent, feeling pressure to perform, having perhaps attempted to satisfy his partner, but to no avail. Somehow he knows he is not reaching her and yet still tries to make the connection through overbearing sexual advances, or gives up completely. Unfortunately, with conventional sex the focus is too much in the area of the genitals, using them to get what is expected and thus leaving out of the picture the whole area of a woman's heart and breasts, the place where her sexual energy is raised. However, as explained in chapter 3, it's in this area that a woman's sexual energy is awakened on a deeper level.

A deep and powerful key for the menopausal woman who wishes to open to her sexuality beyond her middle years lies in cooperating and experimenting with this fundamental difference between male and female bodies. Similarly, conventional sex leaves little time for the movement of energy upward toward the man's receptive pole, his heart. When men at the retreats experience this rise of energy to the heart center, they report that it is the "holy grail" they have been seeking all along.

Creating a Suitable Environment

It's not about learning special techniques; rather we intentionally create an environment in which lovemaking can last longer, allowing the bodies to melt and relax restfully together in deep peace and harmony. It's a conscious choice to create coolness instead of heat. Instead of creating tension through fast movement, friction, and heavy breathing, we go slowly and create relaxation through bringing simple awareness to every moment, which enables the sexual energy to be retained.

It may not seem feasible to the logical mind, but until you have tried it and experienced making love in this way, you cannot easily comprehend the vast world of sensitivity that becomes available to you. Instead of the momentary peak-and-release style of orgasm or ejaculation, the experience of making slow, long love becomes simpler, more spacious, expanded, and blissful, with a peaceful and harmonious quality to it. Having had this blissful experience, going for the orgasm almost becomes a disturbance to the timeless, effortless state of love and pleasure that can arise.

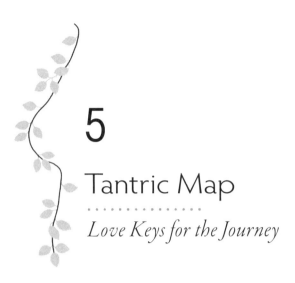

5

Tantric Map

Love Keys for the Journey

BY THE TIME A WOMAN REACHES menopause or perimenopause, she may have been sexually active for at least twenty years, perhaps many more. During this time, much can happen to a woman's body that turns her off sex and makes her shy away from making love, which is the very thing that could offer her a long-lasting connection to her body, her senses, her inner world, and her innate feminine nature.

THE HOW OF SEX

Statistics indicate women's loss of interest in sex is extremely widespread. Countless women report a lifetime of engaging their bodies in sexual activity that has, more often than not, been less than satisfying with no real bonding or connecting. Perhaps a woman has compromised her body for the sake of keeping peace in a relationship, or has done much to avoid sex or get it over with as soon as possible. Alternatively, a woman's wish for sex may be greater than her partner's. Often it's assumed that men want sex more, but there are definitely women who want to have sex more than their men.

On the other hand, a woman may have largely been free to celebrate her own sexuality, yet the passing of years and diminishing of her natural hormones have left her with little interest in sex, while her partner is still very much wanting to engage sexually.

One reason why women feel little hope in the sexual arena is that the way we are doing it, the "how" of sex, is never really questioned. Sex for most couples is comprised of a basic routine done repeatedly over decades; it generally starts the same way each time and always ends the same way each time, with orgasm and ejaculation, which is a peak-and-discharge experience. Additionally there is the reality that many women struggle to have a regular orgasm with penis in vagina; usually it's happening via the clitoris, and for some women that does not do the trick either. The lack of constructive conversation about sex has caused men and women to inadvertently miss out on its higher potential. This next chapter is an in-depth explanation of how to change things.

LOVE KEY 1:
MIND TO BODY

Explained generally to this point, the entire premise of Tantra is about making a shift from mind to body. It is an invitation to become anchored in our physical body in the present moment. However, we cannot think our way into the body. We need to learn to really feel it on a sensing level. And we use our mind to direct awareness into the body—to begin to consciously feel the flesh and bones at any given moment in whatever we are doing, and especially in sex.

In general, the habit is to be "up and out," focused outside of ourselves, so the way to completely transform our experience is to invert our attention and turn "in and down" inside the body. In order to invert the awareness, it is necessary to use the body as a bridge to feeling ourselves in the here and now. And to find a home in there, a place within that feels restful, peaceful, and alive. This could be anywhere that feels sweet, good, and easy to access.

You, First and Foremost

When both individuals consciously drop back into their own bodies before and during sex, there is a natural grounding and disentanglement of projections, and the quality of "being here" can completely transform the experience from ordinary to extraordinary. Frequently we hear from couples in retreats who are putting some of these suggestions into practice, "Wow, we never had such beautiful sex; it's the best ever in my life . . . beyond our wildest dreams." And that feedback comes from both women and men.

Universe of Inner Bodily Sensations

When each person goes in and down, the space between them is cleared of need, cleared of negative tension, cleared of unfulfilled desire. When we are simply present, we are naturally more present to a vast universe of inner bodily sensations we might not have had the chance to notice in the past. With more anchoring in the present we become more inwardly oriented and aligned, and increasingly more observant of the subtle inner movements of the body.

⎘ Opening to the Inner Home

This is a great practice to do on your own. Sit or stand comfortably with a straight spine, and then close your eyes and take your attention into your body. Start to scan your body from head to toe for tensions and, on the out-breath, relax each area you are scanning. With each level of relaxation, go more inward with your attention. Start to bring awareness to how you are sitting or standing, how you are feeling in the body.

Allow your attention to search out a place inside you that feels like "home," a place that is easy for you to feel and inwardly connect with, a place that feels comfortable and easy to access or feel or sense. This settling into yourself can take several minutes, especially if you have been busy before you started the exercise.

Once you have located this inner home, use it as an anchor to your body and the present, continually reminding yourself to fall back into your body and rest with the awareness in your body. If there is no special place that presents itself, just choose one and make that your inner contact point.

After a while you can open your eyes in the receptive way you'll find explained on pages 66–68. When you have practiced accessing your inner home for a while you will find yourself able to access it with eyes open, which makes the practice easy to integrate while engaged in other activities.

Positive Impact on Nervous System

When you scan and relax your body in this way, the whole nervous system relaxes. Relaxing softens the edges. So referring constantly to the body is central to shifting away from the sometimes tense and fractious workings of the mind to being more in the present. The simple exercise given above will help you to be present in the here and now anytime and anywhere, and when applied in lovemaking it creates an energetic space and realm between you and your partner where something can flow and move and dance. It feels very different from when each person is focused more outwardly on the other. With outward focus you can be filled with insecurity and expectation because neither of you is really settled in your own self.

◻ *Opening to Yourself with a Partner*

If you have a partner this practice can be done sitting or standing opposite each other. Begin by closing your eyes and following the process outlined above, each locating an inner home and resting with awareness anchored internally.

After a while you can open your eyes (in the receptive way outlined below). Allow the eyes to meet for a few moments, and then move your bodies across the space into a gentle embrace. Continue to keep your attention on your own body. Now see what happens, how it unfolds, flows, moves. Don't expect anything special, though, because expectation will get in the way of being natural.

LOVE KEY 2:
FROM ABSENCE TO PRESENCE

What feels deeply incongruent for many women, and in particular the menopausal woman, as the receiver of a man's energy, is, as mentioned before, that sex up until now has been relatively unconscious and mechanical. Intentionally building up the heat, tension, and sensation means each is going toward a goal in the future—the event of orgasm and ejaculation. If you are moving toward a goal in sex, you are more focused on achieving a specific event rather than on being anchored in the present. There is a level of aloneness and absence that is inadvertently created within you and between you. Your eyes may be closed as you ride your own sensation and pleasure, without really connecting deeply with yourself or the other. Woman with her heart very near her breasts, her energy-raising area, can easily feel bereft of nourishment by the classic lovemaking scenario and long for connection, instead feeling used. She aches for a man's presence and she aches for her own presence, even though she may not even be aware of what that looks or feels like.

Anchoring in the Body

So how do we create more presence? Presence is a radiance and is the eventual outcome of practicing being more present and body oriented. Being present requires us to be more aware and mindful of whether we are anchored bodily in the unfolding present moment as described above or if we are more focused on striving for a peak, which is considered the goal of sex, the very reason for having sex. To be more aware of our inner experiencing, we need to first start to observe ourselves as individuals and become aware of how easily we get ahead of ourselves, and usually we are aiming to create a peak. When it comes to lovemaking, often our level of presence is affected by wondering if the other is okay, what the other is thinking or feeling, or whether we or they are doing it "right."

This goal-oriented pattern means we are constantly absent and there is a lack of connection to the present moment that can be subtly felt by the other. This habit of being goal focused also has an effect on the body because our thoughts form an energetic overlay on our bodies, making them less relaxed and open, and more contracted and rigid.

LOVE KEY 3:
FROM SENSATION TO SENSITIVITY

The question then is how do we become more sensitive to ourselves and to the other? It's important to understand that high sensation and intensity can cause an ultimately dulling effect, a dampening effect on the whole body and psyche. This is nowhere better illustrated than in the current trend of men and boys watching internet porn and carrying over its negative effects into their bodies in response to real women in real-life situations. If they are engaging in a lot of porn, men can become numb to the real thing and find they are unable to get or sustain an erection in real life, due to the high, fast sensation kick from porn.

Sadly, the more we engage in sensation, the more insensitive the body becomes. This numbness in turn can cause a craving for more sensation, and with this additional sensation, increasingly and correspondingly less sensitivity will be experienced. It's a bit of a vicious circle. In addition to boys using porn, more and more young women are as well. There is a whole body of science that shows the hormonal effects on the brain and why this is so damaging to the sensitivity of body and mind.

An article by Belinda Luscombe in *Time* magazine examines porn and its effects in great depth. She writes:

A growing number of young men are convinced that their sexual responses have been sabotaged because their brains were virtually marinated in porn when adolescents. . . . And compelling new research on visual stimuli is offering some support to the young men's theories—a disconnect between what they wanted in the mind (i.e. to have sex with a woman) and how the body reacted—

suggesting the combination of computer access, sexual pleasure, and the brain's mechanisms for learning could make online porn acutely habit forming, with potential psychological effects. In the state of Utah the legislature unanimously passed a resolution to treat pornography as a public health crisis. Gary Wilson, author of *Your Brain on Porn: Internet Pornography and the Emerging Science of Addiction,* supports the link between heavy adolescent pornography use and sexual dysfunction.*

Habits adopted as a young man continue into a man's adult life for decades, which will then have an impact on his relationship with women as he gets older and, if he has a partner, as she becomes menopausal. Effectively the brain has the capacity and plasticity to rewire itself once repeated stimulation and intensity is dramatically reduced. The same is true for the female body. You may not even notice if your vagina has lost its sensitivity, but the good news is that sensitivity can be regained. And the same goes for men. So it helps to make a shift from high sensation, which creates absence through being focused on intensity, to sensitivity where you feel yourself in the moment, which creates presence.

Challenge Desire for Sensation

When a woman does not have a lot of evident physical sexual response, it can be very tempting for her to seek sensation, even at a subtle level, just to prove to herself that there is nothing wrong with her, that her body does work, that she can feel. Often, however, it can seem to be such hard work to feel that ultimately she gives up trying. But if she and her partner can be patient, and be in there for the long haul, they both will find treasures along the way. All of a sudden energy spreads and sweetens throughout the body; the feeling of union comes in unex-

---

*Belinda Luscombe, *Time* (April 11, 2016), 34; and Gary Wilson, *Your Brain on Porn: Internet Pornography and the Emerging Science of Addiction* (Margate, Kent, U.K.: Commonwealth Publishing, 2015).

pected surprises, especially when you are not looking for anything in particular. Not being goal oriented, not seeking, just creating the space will reward you a hundred times over.

Hot to Cool

Conventional sex draws us into a pattern of seeking more and more sensation by making it hotter and hotter. Consider that something hot will always, of necessity, cool down; you cannot stay hot forever. While "hot" can be exciting and even exhilarating, it is a momentary experience.

In Tantra we are looking to something that is sustainable and lasting that will stay with us beyond the actual event of sex. So it helps to combine the Love Keys* to be more present by staying with the body, to be interested in sensitivity, *and* to remain conscious of how hot—or not—we are getting in lovemaking.

Because something hot is not long lasting, the natural tendency is to look for ways to make things even more exciting. So the search is basically to get hotter and hotter, finding more sensation through sex toys, new partners, or pornography while making love.

If a woman at this stage of her life has not engaged in anything like that up until now, she may also be tempted down the sensation track, especially if she feels she needs revving up to get her body going because there seems to be little response. Added to that, a new kind of liberation may lure her there to experience things that were once taboo in her world. Indeed, these may bring excitement and fulfill something for the moment but in the end will more likely lead her to a dead end. Such expeirence can in fact create more distance from the body, because she is predominantly inhabiting the mind and using the imagination.

To move from hot to a cooler approach might be quite challenging

---

*These Love Keys and guidelines were initially elaborated in Diana Richardson's first book, written in 1996, initially entitled *The Love Keys, the Art of Ecstatic Sex: A Unique Guide to Love and Sexual Fulfillment,* and then republished under its current title *The Heart of Tantric Sex: A Unique Guide to Love and Sexual Fulfillment* (Arlesford, Hants, U.K.: "O" Books, 2010).

for men; however, for the menopausal woman, it is sheer luxury. Finally she is able to relish lovemaking in relaxing, in being, instead of racing to get somewhere. She is now taking the space to open in her own time. And when man supports woman and understands her body is different and she needs more time before he enters her, he finds himself in a totally different universe, abundantly rewarded by the flowering and showering of love he receives from his woman.

LOVE KEY 4: RECEPTIVE EYES

The eyes are said to be the windows of the soul, yet looking and seeing can be two different things. We are accustomed to going about our lives not even aware of the gift of sight, taking it for granted. Again, we are always looking outward. Our attention and energy is projected outward making an effort "to see," whereas the eyes are designed to receive images with no real effort required on our part.

Receiving through the Eyes

In Tantra we suggest again to invert the energy of "looking outward" through the eyes and instead "receiving" what you are seeing. Rather than looking out, allow the image to come to you. Again the inverted gaze rather than the extroverted gaze—one of receiving your partner into your space, your world, rather than actively looking—creates a totally different quality of seeing. You are opening to one of your major senses and allowing the other in on another level. It is not in any way happening as an invasion, rather it is as if you are inviting the other person in.

Through this process you will naturally soften your eyes; they suddenly become more relaxed and less judgmental and critical and they appear softer to others too. When you consciously practice inverting your vision, an energetic exchange arises without having to make something happen. Love flows and spontaneously you relax and smile.

One Eye at a Time

If you attempt to "receive" both eyes at once, it can have a mesmerizing effect. So it's best to connect with one eye rather than attempt both at the same time. Also avoid repeatedly switching your eyes rapidly from one to the other; stay with one eye for a while, and then if you wish, move to the other. Once you have settled in and down into yourself, then open your eyes: viewing the other from this receptive place transforms what and how you see.

If your eyes get tired, close them to relax and then open again when you feel ready. It's good to let the other person know, in words or gestures, that you are just closing them for a short time to reconnect with yourself. Communicate that you will return soon! If you open your eyes and your partner's eyes happen to be closed, simply receive your partner's face with love.

◌ Receptive Vision in Nature

It does take time to get the knack of this sort of seeing and the very best way of playing with receiving through the eyes is in nature. Any time you come across a beautiful view, sunset, tree, or flower, stop moving, stand still, and anchor yourself inwardly as described in the exercise on pages 60–61. Once you feel internally settled, begin to open your eyes extremely slowly, millimeter by millimeter. Let the eyes open about halfway (not fully) and keep them receptively soft, maintaining your attention in your body, and imagine that the view, that the beauty, is reaching or flowing toward you and you are receiving it through your eyes. Then allow it to enter you and to touch you. When you get the feel of this way of visually receiving, you can begin to open the eyes fully, and not just halfway. Having them half-open makes it easier, in the beginning, to establish that sense of receiving, of absorbing through the eyes. This sounds almost too simple, but it is extremely effective. Interestingly, artists who use this way of seeing paint a very different type of picture.

◻ *Practice Receptive Vision with a Partner*

If you have a partner it's great to try this way of seeing with each other. Begin with each of you in your own space, either sitting or standing opposite each other. Start by closing your eyes and following the process outlined in the exercise on pages 60–61, with each locating an inner home and resting with awareness anchored internally. After a while you can open your eyes in the receptive way outlined above, bring them to the face of your partner, and allow the eyes to meet for a few moments. Important is to notice if you lose contact with your inner body. If you do, close your eyes again and reanchor yourself internally. When you feel ready, open your eyes again. It does require practice to develop this way of seeing, so be patient with yourself and also practice in nature, whenever possible.

LOVE KEY 5:
BREATH

If we do not breathe, we die. Yet so much of our fast-paced lifestyle compromises our breathing without our even being aware of it. If you take the time to just sit quietly and feel your natural breathing, you might find that it is indeed a little shallow and uses only part of the lungs, often just the upper part. This dulls our senses and makes us feel less than alive and vital.

Breath Revitalizes

Breath will inject greater life force into your experience, not only in your daily life, but also while making love. As you breathe you recharge and enliven the cells within the body. It also deeply relaxes the entire system and generates sexual energy that then moves and expands throughout your body to create more fluidity and aliveness.

Draw the Breath Down to the Genitals

If you sit and breathe with intention and awareness, breathing down-ward in the direction of the genitals and the lower pelvic area, and open yourself to your breath, you will notice that it creates a lovely rhythm within the body. It increases relaxation and allows you to fall back into yourself more deeply. As you breathe you will be more aware of your chest and breasts, and the gentle rhythm as they rise and fall allows you to open to the subtle energy within the body and tap into the inner rod of magnetism (as explained in chapter 3). You may also feel some resonance within the vagina, or perhaps in the womb area.

Breath Increases Body Connection

The breath is a beautiful bridge to your body—it's the way back home. If you feel that your mind has run away mid–making love, breath will bring you back in just an instant. Breath plus awareness equals actual experience of the present moment. Use conscious breathing often in lovemaking (and daily life) as an anchor to yourself, especially when you feel as if you are focusing too much on the other person. A simple breath will glide you effortlessly back into yourself. It will transform your whole experience of being in your body and being with another.

Slow and Deep Breathing

It's good to breathe deeply and slowly. Just be careful to not make it a heavy "dragon breath." Keep the breathing deep but light, like a feather gently touching the surface of the ocean. This deeper breathing will also enable you to keep the sexual atmosphere cooler, so as not to generate too much heat that can so easily lead to peak and discharge.

LOVE KEY 6:
STROKING AND CARESSING

The body has nerve endings radiating all over it, and a woman's body is especially sensitive. If you compress and push on or squeeze someone's body, that pressure suppresses the more delicate and fine level of sensing and feeling in the tissues (sometimes called the "felt sense," or kinesthetic sense) and causes a kind of dullness or numbness. For example, if someone hugs you and squeezes your body too tight, you end up feeling the other person and not really able to feel yourself at all.

Porousness

If you keep the touch light and porous, rather than firm and dense, there is space for expansion of the invisible energy body that surrounds it. Imagine that the edges of your skin and body are not finite, that your flesh is in fact made up of millions of moving, vibrant cells, the very force of life itself.

Thus when you are entering the energy field of another's body, it is sensitive and sacred. When you bring this quality of porousness or lightness or delicateness to your touch, you will feel the difference, and your partner will as well. Your sensitivity naturally increases, your body sparkles with light. You become conscious in each moment of the touch rather than repeating movements that are mechanical or rough.

In the same way, approaching the kiss can be met without pressing or forcing, but it can be very sensual with a spacious, yet fully engaged, meeting of the lips. We suggest that you explore the whole terrain of the lips, avoiding getting too hot through tongue kissing if you wish to stay in the cooler zone.

Include the Whole Body

Remember to touch the whole body and not just one area, for women adore being touched all over the body. Best is to begin by caressing and stroking the extremities until we are longing or wishing for the touch to extend toward our breasts and genitals. Men also delight in their bodies being given conscious, loving attention.

Touching the Breasts

The touching of the breasts is something that is best for you to communicate with your partner first, explaining how you like it done—what works and doesn't work for you. Also bear in mind that it's not a fixed route, each meeting is unique, plus every woman is so different with her sensitivity and with her history. The idea is to open to your breasts from within—it is not about creating stimulation or excitement.

That is why it's good to take time with yourself in front of the mirror or in your own space and touch and hold your breasts, learning to feel yourself first before being with the other. Then you know from the inside to what and how your body responds. Men are often left guessing, but they are usually very good at wanting to please you and therefore often happy to take directions if you guide them. So take advantage of that! Usually the simple cupping and holding of a woman's breasts will be adequate for her. Also worth experimenting with is when a woman is sitting or standing and her man is embracing her from behind, and holding her breasts. This is very comforting and really helps a woman open to her breasts and feel herself.

Touching the Penis and Testicles

Similarly, it's good to ask your partner how and where he likes to be touched. Most men really enjoy having their penises touched in a relaxed, loving way, giving a gentle massage instead of trying to stimulate. Each man is different, so open up a conversation. Make sure to stay in awareness and keep the touch simple, without mechanical rubbing, sending your love into the penis or holding and connecting with it—in a nondemanding and nonstimulating way.

LOVE KEY 7:
RELAXATION

Knowing you want to relax and actually managing to do so are two entirely different things, but certain awareness practices can be very supportive.

Body Scanning

All of what we have said so far invites relaxation on many different levels. In addition, consciously scanning the whole body for tension is a great way to bring awareness to places where you are holding uncon-sciously, and then to soften to find a place of relaxation. After the con-scious relaxation of any body part, a deep and grateful breath generally will follow in response. And if you are alert, you will notice an expan-sion of subtle good feelings inside the body. You may not even be aware there is any tension until you experience pain, and then it can take quite a lot of awareness and unwinding to reach a place of relaxation.

Relax the Genital Area

In order to bring your body to a more sparkling, alive, awake state in your daily life or during lovemaking, it helps enormously to consciously relax any genital tightness. And you will notice how much better you feel in your body. Scan the genitals and the pelvic floor with your awareness again and again. It may seem counterintuitive to think you can relax your genitals, or even that there might be tension there, but it's very true. The genital area of both men and women can carry a lot of tension, especially as most of us are subtly contracting the pelvic floor on an ongoing basis without even noticing. In men, there can be tension in the buttocks, anus, pelvic floor, penis, testicles, and the groin area. In women tension can be found in the vagina, its surrounding tis-sues, and generally the whole pelvic floor and pelvic region. Women are especially likely to hold tension in the pelvis because there are many ligaments that elegantly hold her pelvic organs and support the uterus, especially for possible pregnancy. (Refer to chapter 11 for further read-ing on abdominal healing.)

Your body will directly respond to your intention to relax specific areas, and when you scan for tensions repeatedly, you will notice how this awareness will spread throughout your body and bring the cells into an alive, vibrant place. They "hear" and somehow respond. The cells exist as pure consciousness and sensing your inner connection at this level will absolutely change the quality of your genital experience.

Consciousness simply is. That is the mystery of the universe and of life. Consciousness is the vitality of every single cell, a vast innate intelligence in every fiber of the human body right down to the molecular structure. Each hand is filled with consciousness. Each leg is filled with consciousness. Mind-body medicine is proving this now not only through science; memories are spontaneously surfacing from harvested donor body parts put into another body via organ donation. So the genitals are filled with their very own consciousness and intelligence, and bringing our awareness to this level means we are accessing new aliveness and sensitivity, empowering the body with life force.

Vagina Designed to Receive

Tantra honors equally the feminine force and the masculine force, and this understanding extends to the level of the genitals. Male genitals are external and the protruding male penis is a conduit for the dynamic force that moves toward the receptive, of its own accord, and without "doing" anything. The vagina, the internal portion of the female genitals, is designed to receive and absorb this dynamic force. Receptivity in itself is a force and power. It does not mean passivity or submissiveness, tameness, or meekness. In truth, the intrinsic dynamic flow of male energy can only come into being when there is a corresponding spaciousness of the receptive female force.

Even procreation illustrates this; the egg, released from the ovary, waits inside the uterus to be impregnated by the sperm. The female creates the environment and produces the hormones to attract it. The sperm from the male is the moving force that seeks out the egg and penetrates it to produce life.

Relax the Vagina to Increase Receptivity

Just knowing that the vagina is a receptor—a space to soften, relax, and expand—can give a woman enormous confidence.

When a woman perceives her vagina as a receptive pole, she can open herself to truly receiving the penis in love. And it's highly likely she will feel as if she is absorbing the dynamic force of the penis in a relaxed, innocent, and conscious way. She no longer has to "make something happen" within her vagina, as the awareness she brings into the tissues and cells creates its very own powerful environment. This quality of receptivity heightens and transforms the energetic exchange between penis and vagina and a new frontier of experience becomes available to us.

Recalibrating the Vagina

When the vagina is more receptive, the dynamic energy emanating from the penis truly has somewhere to move and flow. Despite whatever friction and tension may have been experienced in the past, relaxation enables the vagina to soften, open, and recalibrate to become the absorbing, receptive organ nature designed it to be.

Awareness on Base of Penis

Likewise, a man can bring his attention to the root of the penis, focusing more on the base in the area of the perineum, rather than on the tip, and he will find this awareness changes the quality of his lovemaking and his presence in general. It will help him to be less "doing" in sex, and thereby gain access to the love residing inside of him; something he yearns for, often unknowingly. Many men have shared this in our couples groups. Genital awareness brings a heightened sensitivity that is far more enduring and relaxing, and through this lovemaking can last for hours. This is good news for the perimenopausal and menopausal woman and her partner, because no longer is repetitive friction needed as the only option for sexual exchange. New vistas may open beyond anything ever experienced or explored previously.

LOVE KEY 8:
CONSCIOUS MOVEMENT

Life is movement. Even in apparent stillness there is movement. A leaf on a tree that appears still can be moving to a micro degree, affected by the breeze and light around it. So it is with the body. In conventional sex there is generally a lot of external movement needed to sustain excitement and to achieve the desired orgasm and ejaculation. Tantra invites us to bring more awareness to movement, to be conscious in any movement. And in the very simple act of awareness an entire universe of sensitivity is revealed.

For example, if you go on a walk with the intention of being more conscious of every step you take and what you see around you, you will notice yourself naturally moving more slowly. You will have more awareness of the colors and shapes of your surroundings, the feel of the ground beneath your feet, the light, perhaps others passing by, the temperature of the air. You are much more available to your surroundings and thus you can be more receptive to how that touches you or not. You may even be uplifted by your ability to feel more; a sense of brightness may come over you and a lightness of being.

Conscious Leads to Slow

When we direct our awareness inward during lovemaking, we notice that quite naturally, through being conscious, we tend to slow our movements. And through that, there is a resulting slowness, increasing sensitivity. We actually feel more.

You will both be more available to the slightest nuance, as the sweet fragrance of love embraces you. This slowness and amplification of the senses for a menopausal woman, in fact any woman regardless of age, is tantalizing. She comes alive through slowness; her body naturally and gracefully responds. She can feel more, rather than have her senses compressed by friction or mechanical movements.

In the same way, man has more time to experience himself on another level. He can begin to open to a world of sensitivity he may not have felt before, with the sexual energy moving gently in waves toward his heart. Sometimes he may experience a huge relief, as he no longer has the pressure of performing and getting it right. Some tears may even arise, probably as a release of the accumulated tension due to performance stress.

The two bodies begin to move effortlessly together in a wave-like rhythm, somewhat like a small boat being tipped gently and rhythmically by a warm embracing sea. When you can be totally present with the aliveness and vitality within and between you, the hearts naturally connect and the bodies become even more fluid and more finely attuned.

Stillness

If you can let go (of the control) and let your body organically just "do its own thing," you may find that it comes to a place of outer stillness. But this stillness is not a boring, inert stillness. Stillness in conventional sex is what usually marks the end of lovemaking after the peak, when the penis has relaxed and there is no more physical movement. However, stillness in Tantra is a profound, timeless stillness; a dynamic stillness that pulses with life and life force. You may feel the circulation of sexual energy palpably or not. A pulsing may even start to be felt in the genitals or sometimes for a woman in the womb area, the lower pelvic region, or even the whole body. This stillness has a vibrant, expansive, and blissful quality to it.

Relax When No Erection

It can take time for a man to become used to lovemaking in a more relaxed style, as his sexual conditioning to "do" something in sex is deeply rooted. At times he may feel his erection go down due to less friction and stimulating movement. He may become anxious and insecure that his erection is receding. However, with his intention to stay present, he can relax, and with a little bit of slow, conscious movement the erection is likely to return. And if it doesn't, just enjoy the presence of the penis resting in the vagina, and being simply together. Sometimes, in this relaxed state and even without movement, the erection may unexpectedly begin to grow, spiraling into the vagina, as if the genitals are making love by themselves. The energy exchange occurs organically and magnetically and does not involve technique or goal-oriented intentions. It's quite a feeling! This spontaneous erection within the vagina is extraordinary and practically unheard of in conventional sex. We believe we need to do something, because there is a fear of not feeling anything or that nothing is going to happen unless we make an effort.

But once we start to relax and just be present in the here and now, the bodies can take over perfectly. It's especially good for women to know that where their attention is placed dramatically influences the dynamics of the energy exchange. If the woman is a bit distracted and thinking of something else, such as a problem at work or a household task, the spontaneous erection will surely subside. So for her to directly return her attention to being anchored and present in her body will bring her, and him, back beautifully. Gentle movement can also help, or a shift in position. And if this does not have an effect, appreciate the exchange for what it is, because even without erection there is something happening. In time, when this subtle energy exchange is given value, erections cease to have the overriding importance they do in conventional sex. It used to be more common that men over fifty had issues with erection, but now it seems to be affecting younger and younger men, primarily related to high levels of sensation in sex, now exacerbated by pornography as mentioned earlier. If a man is willing to be patient and pass through this phase of not feeling much, he will notice, over time, even after just a few lovemaking sessions, that his sensitivity will indeed gradually return.

Feelings Can Rise to the Surface

Sometimes slowing things down can be quite confronting, because with more awareness, strong feelings can arise—tears, sadness, or grief from the past, or uplifting feelings of gratitude, love, and deep appreciation. All these expressions are totally okay and can be welcomed with understanding. Share with your partner what you are feeling, and for the one listening, there's no need to try to fix or change the situation. Just listen, be present, and be supportive of the old feelings arising for your partner. Allowing these previously unexpressed feelings creates intimacy and bonding, and also cleanses and purifies the whole system.

PATIENCE IS A FRIEND ON THE JOURNEY

Any time we are embarking on unknown territory, patience is required to establish ourselves comfortably on the journey. Often menopausal women have not made love for a while, therefore there is quite a bit of insecurity that requires patience and understanding. At times we may judge ourselves for not doing it "right," but there is *no* right or wrong in the whole experience. It's best to have the attitude of explorers and an attitude of innocence. Sometimes you might go off track, as in going for the peak of orgasm; if that happens, relax and enjoy it fully! Or experiment with being more relaxed in the body and vagina as you go into orgasm.

Tools Not Rules

These Love Keys are suggestions and tools, never rules. When we have rules about something, we become rigid and linear in our thinking, and that translates to narrowing and compression in our bodies. Bodies become tense, hard, and closed with rules, self-imposed or otherwise. This is not Tantra. Tantra means and implies expansion—like opening to the vastness of the sky. So relax and remember there is no right or wrong. See it as a series of experiments, and this attitude will support you in moving forward. Also, if you resist orgasm this will create tension too. And we wish to remove tension in all ways, so go with it and allow and just notice how you feel afterward.

Afterward Informs You

In fact, how you feel afterward as you go about your daily life is definitely a reference point. Afterward teaches and informs you, and can be the most interesting and revealing inquiry. If you feel a deep contentment in your being afterward, a relaxation not quite felt before, a sweet feeling of the tendrils of love inside you, then take note of how your lovemaking was. It may not even have been spectacular or memorable, but more often than not, we have definitely noticed that lovemaking in awareness, relaxation, and sensitivity is followed by contented, fulfilled feelings.

And also observe, as we have done, that if there has been tension and climactic orgasm and ejaculation, afterward very often there can be a feeling of disconnection or sense of separation. Many couples deny experiencing this when we first mention it, but then when they begin to bring their attention to this aspect, most report remembering that in fact this is how they have felt for years. They thought it was a normal part of sex. Following the peak and discharge, there has always been a feeling of slight emptiness, flatness, depression, withdrawal, and disconnection. Even flashes of anger or low-level frustration have popped up at times. And be aware that negative effects can be felt or observed some days later.*

When couples in our seven-day Making Love Retreats decide intentionally to go for a peak, they definitely observe that the beautiful, sweet, connected feelings of love that were palpably there previously—created over several days through being aware and present while having sex—seem to disappear and evaporate immediately after the peak. This occurs in particular when the man ejaculates. This is definitely not to say never to allow orgasm and ejaculation, just to be aware of how you feel afterward, and to take note. This is an inquiry that challenges sexual patterns and habits of lifetimes and this is also why you need to have patience. When you have the inner observer on board, you can make choices for the future regarding how cool you wish to keep lovemaking, or how you deal with any emotions and feelings should they arise afterward, as explained in chapter 10.

---

*This subject is elaborated upon by the scientific research presented in Marnia Robinson's book *Cupid's Poisoned Arrow*. See recommended books section.

FOR SINGLE WOMEN

If you are single you have a beautiful opportunity to tune your body to the flow of the natural energy inherent within it, without the disturbance of another.

Ecstasy Lies within You

Whether or not you have a partner you can engage with yourself fully, and that is a blessing. It's time now to really recognize and accept that these fine fulfilling and delicate energies exist within you, and you do not need a partner. Connecting with yourself inwardly through any of the guidelines and suggested exercises in this book can be an empowering practice of becoming attuned to your delicate and fine sensitivity. Later on this awareness will have an impact on your life in general, and if you do meet a partner in the future, it will enhance your sexual experience and amplify love between you.

Self-Pleasuring (Masturbation)

The same guideline applies for self-pleasure—you bring awareness to the inner experience and notice what that is like. Notice what you are doing and how you are doing it. The tendency is to focus outside the vagina and on the clitoris for direct pleasure. A woman can start to become aroused very quickly and fall into the convention—fast, hot friction that is over very quickly. We suggest you take the time to notice how it leaves you feeling afterward. Even though it feels good in the moment, perhaps you notice you become a bit negative, edgy, angry, irritable, or sad. And as already mentioned, sometimes negativity can manifest several days down the track, not only in the period immediately following the event.

However, loving your own body through sensitive, slow touch and sensual caressing is a beautiful act of self-love and allows you to get in tune with your own likes and dislikes, to come to know your own body more intimately. You can experiment with caressing and stroking your body in an upward motion that encourages expansion of energy and sensitivity. Self-loving in this way gives you permission to feel that your body is for you and your own pleasure. And for women who have always "done it for another," this can be quite enlivening.

If you do wish to come to the peak of orgasm, imagine falling back into yourself, relaxing and widening, allowing the waves to come on their own without having to work for it. And if it does not come, notice how that feels, if there is some disappointment. Of course, if you choose not to orgasm, consciously allow the vitality to spread through your body. You will feel lusciously feminine and this quality will exude from you like the fragrance of a beautiful flower in the summer heat.

So we suggest that masturbation is an option to be used only occasionally. Due to the fact that tensions are inadvertently created, it's not something we suggest you do regularly. More refreshing for you will be to open to the feelings of bliss inherent within the body and allow them to expand without the need to do anything with them or taking sensations in a specific direction. We discover and learn to be more present and less goal-oriented. Sometimes the urge to masturbate in order to have an orgasm is a reflection of other tensions and stresses of life. It's an easy way to off-load. However, it can leave one feeling ungrounded, empty, and nervous, especially if done on a regular or habitual basis. We have had many reports from women who were quite dependent on stimulation of the clitoris during sex or masturbation, but then tried staying away from it and containing the energy instead, saying how much better they felt, more grounded emotionally, more stable, and on an even keel.

DIFFICULTY WITH ORGASM

Many women who attend our retreats report never having had an orgasm. Others say that they struggle to bring themselves to a peak, only managing it occasionally. There are a number of reasons why this can be so; for example, because a woman's body has not been deeply awakened or because the sex act is usually over very quickly due to premature male ejaculation. When we consider the negative effects of peak orgasms, as described above, with the physical tension and intensity required to "get there," it is of great value for women to question, is "it" really and truly worth it? For all women in general, and in particular those women who struggle with orgasm, there is an urgent need to reevaluate our ingrained belief that the orgasm is what sex is basically about. Our sexual conditioning has invested our psyches in wanting peak orgasms to the extent that a woman will begin to doubt herself and not feel like a full-blooded woman unless she can have an orgasm. This is terribly sad, because the peak orgasm is essentially meaningless on a deeper energetic level—it is usually a downward flow of energy that leaks tensions in the system. And then afterward there are frequently feelings of abandonment, emptiness, disconnection, or sadness. Of course this may not be the case every single time, but it is good to pay attention to the guideline that "afterward is your teacher" and keep track of yourself over several months. Of greater value for woman is discovering her God-given orgasmic nature, and developing the capacity to contain and circulate energy within. And to realize that through becoming one with her breasts she will invite her deepest orgasmic experiences, and these will be much more enriching and life enhancing.

What Diana Remembers

Once a woman in Brazil told me that when she was younger she had a wonderful sex life, even though she never ever had orgasms. Even so, she was totally happy and content until one day unexpectedly she had one! And she said that from that day onward her sex life went downhill. She kept trying to repeat that same experience again and again. She got totally tense in body and mind trying to reach her new goal. This personal story reveals how strong the hold of the psyche and the mind over the body can be. It also indicates that we need to free ourselves of ideas, concepts, and goals that interfere with the joyful and relaxed celebration of our bodies in the present.

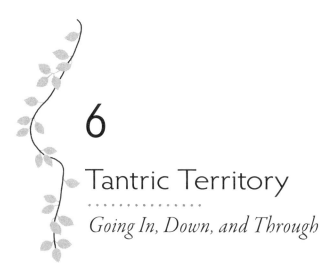

6

Tantric Territory

Going In, Down, and Through

UNTIL ABOUT TWO HUNDRED YEARS AGO, many women did not live beyond age forty. Women were often pregnant almost every year and therefore were perhaps never confronted by how menopause manifested in their lives. Many others died in childbirth. The wonders of modern-day medicine have prolonged our lives so that a woman can now live to twice that age or older. For those who do, the process of menopause is inescapable. The body ages, fertility wanes, and changes occur. A woman either handles it gracefully or it handles her. She can't ignore it; if she resists, the body catches up with her anyway. It can take her down into the deep waters of her own psyche, into the undergrowth of her life. It unearths. It sheds. It renews . . . if she lets it.

Janet remembers her revelation:

While I was in the thick of perimenopause, all I remember thinking was I wanted to be "put out to pasture," to be left alone, or to bury myself deep under the earth. Not to die, but to renew. I felt like I was living a Greek myth, caught in some futuristic life in the twenty-first century yet on the inside being invited into a mythical underworld. When I contemplate the meaning of these feelings, what I get is that one calling was for deep rest of the body; the other was for deep wisdom of the soul. There was nothing I could do with my mind—it all had to be done to me, to my psyche. I had to allow it. It felt very archetypal. I wanted to paint, to write, to create. And for no one to ask anything of me.

ACCEPTANCE OF CHANGE
IS THE WAY FORWARD

Like birth and puberty, nothing happens overnight. There is always a transition stage from a growing fetus to the birth of a child, a girl transitioning into a woman, and now midlife woman walking through the portal into her elder life. In this stage a woman may feel herself to be in some kind of nowhere land. It might feel like she is treading muddy waters or facing a vast wasteland, depending on her life situation. There may be physical symptoms dragging her down emotionally, sleep may be difficult, and anger may lurk just below the surface. The way she has been in the past doesn't work for her anymore, yet a new way of being hasn't yet made itself apparent to her. There's an urgency to be left alone and to move onward in her life.

Yet just as in pregnancy birth cannot be forced, the transition of menopause needs time to gestate inside the womb of your psyche, the womb of existence. All resistance creates tension, so if you want to relax, practicing an attitude of acceptance is the way. Yes, it is okay. Naturally when change is upon us a part of us resists, especially if the onset of menopause is sudden or unexpected. For some women menopause is brought on by surgery or an illness that has caused removal of the womb and ovaries. Sometimes a woman goes into menopause when she thought she might still be able to bear a child.

Whatever meaning the onset of menopause has for a woman, tension and unhappiness will accumulate if she is not willing to symbolically go in, down, and through the process. For many women menopause is a watershed of all that was not expressed or consciously felt previously—the deepest fears, the deepest grievances, or the deepest rage. Primal feelings spill into everyday circumstances. Just as in the time prior to menstruation emotions can be immensely heightened, menopause is often a time of purging of what was denied, hidden, or ignored—the too-early death of a parent, sexual boundaries being crossed, the deep grief of your first love, the loss of babies through choice or circumstance, the rage of injustice in a relationship, or even what is happening on a worldwide scale. It could be anything that had been shelved for another day.

To ignore these stored emotions (our unexpressed feelings) can initiate a downward spiral of deep unhappiness and perhaps even bitterness that leave you feeling like a victim of circumstance. Yet to meet and embrace these old feelings can open you to a whole new level of living. As feelings that arise in the present, they must be honored and allowed to move through you. They eventually will let go of you if you accept them and give them space. It's not necessary to try to figure out their source. If you know, you know, and if you don't know, there is absolutely no need to understand why this release is happening. Sometimes in the process you might have an insight or see a picture that perhaps indicates the root of the old feelings, but these insights come spontaneously and don't need to be consciously sought. Trust the situation and relax into the healing opportunity presented, understanding that awareness brought into the body has purifying effects. And if some themes are continually recurring, then you might want to consider receiving professional support.

For Janet, her biggest struggle with early menopause was with the loss of her fertility:

When my periods started to falter and fade away around age forty-one, I went into deep grief at the loss of my ability to conceive. I already had two beautiful children and knew I did not want another child, but there was this primal drive that rose up inside of me. Because it felt too early for me, I cried rivers of sadness letting go of what I had considered to be the ultimate symbol of womanhood— the ability to bear a child. I cried for the children I never had, for the children I could have had. And finally one day it all settled. And there was acceptance and I could move on.

Menopause is a time of folding inward to the source. It calls a woman to go within, and its pull cannot be ignored. A woman may have been outwardly oriented all her life in the corporate or business world, actively parenting, and involved in her community. Now her hormones are drawing her back inward, back home, to stay in her home, her center. It's a call she cannot ignore. Among indigenous peoples and in times past when civilizations lived in community, the women spent their time together doing their tasks, and men were together doing their tasks for much of the day. Outside of the work environment we now are separated into individual dwellings of mostly just two adults, or perhaps alone.

Sometimes we simply need to be with other women—to cry, to feel, to move through our personal experiences. To go in, down, and through together can be a balm for a woman's soul, so that we support each other to move beyond our self-imposed limits.

A NEW PARTNERSHIP WITH YOURSELF

This is a time for woman to start to put herself first (including sexually) and to challenge the conditioning to please, serve, make others happy, and give beyond her physical and emotional ability to do so anymore. This is often when a woman feels selfish, but the miracle of it all is that when she starts first with herself, instead of everyone else, she can start to fill her own cup. With the light of awareness, she can begin to rest in her being, be her own soul, feel her own heart from within, and nourish her body. When she is contacting a much more real and authentic part of herself, she has so much more to give, and this very giving opens the channel for her to receive.

Trust Your Body
Self-love is something beyond pampering the body and getting a massage, though that can certainly help in many cases. It is something far

wilder and far more intuitive. Trusting the deeper messages from the body and the heart, and having the courage to follow, will lead you to greater inner love. The need for a woman to go more slowly in her life emerges as a deep intuitive knowing as much as a necessity. When her body symptoms, life circumstances, or illness stop her in her tracks, her body calls her to respond differently. And the same goes for making love. Where previously she might have gritted her teeth and gotten through, as one woman once described it, now there's simply no desire to push through, no inclination, almost a sense of "couldn't be bothered" where before there was a can-do attitude.

Her instinctive inclination now is to hold the energy within, to not seek the excitement of the outside world anymore, to not expel that energy in unnecessary, unfulfilling experiences. Her soul is calling her to dive down, bed down, and just be. She is not bothered to sit in on conversations that have little meaning, or waste time on relationships that lack depth. Her wild soul is deeply calling her into the vastness of love. Instead of the potential to birth babies, she is now free to birth herself into a new life. It's an exciting pilgrimage that can only be taken alone, while inviting the support of trusted others.

Challenging the desire to fulfill another's needs, not just in the bedroom but in all of life, is a shift for many women, but it is such a worthwhile endeavor, rewarding beyond your imagination. Entering your body with awareness and connecting with the richness of your "inner body" brings a new lover onto the scene, a new partnership— the partnership with self! An empty cup has nothing to give or offer, but filled with the radiance of your own love, you definitely have something to give and share. So start with yourself and your own body, directing awareness into it as an ongoing practice during daily activities, and also while at rest. And even if you have a partner, your own body is nonetheless the priority when you move into any physical exchange. Prepare the body. Move it. Discover what gives you joy inside, in being on your own, instead of expecting another to give you that. Joy and love go hand in hand.

Making Love as Medicine

If you have a partner, making love in awareness and relaxation can be the most beautiful antidote for the menopausal woman. Using the guidelines from the previous chapter and creating more presence between partners seems to induce a level of timelessness that takes lovers into a primordial space where a woman can receive the deep rest she is craving (and a man can discover a way to be engaged in sex in a relaxed way). She does not have to go out to find the rest. Rest is intrinsic to the simple act of receiving and relaxing into being while making love. In this way her body is replenished and feels rejuvenated. She develops a new zest for life, a new courage to gather her wisdom and live more fully. When she experiences how love can begin within her and ripple outward, she can find a peace inside herself that she may have been seeking for her entire life.

These experiences are profoundly life changing, as they change the very cells of your body and touch your being. Transformation happens for both men and women. Words cannot even describe the connection and depth of love available. It is profound. Because hormones do not drive the menopausal woman so much anymore, a woman's ability and capacity to open into a silent, restful state is greatly amplified. For a man to experience making love with the menopausal woman means that he will, if she has surrendered authentically to accepting her body changes, receive the gift of silence and sensitivity he may never before have encountered. This transforms him as he experiences a deep relief inside his body with not having to do so much, just learning to relax and be, and so balancing his body, heart, and soul.

♂ Attuning to Love

Sit still and place your hand over your heart. Breathe in and out with awareness. Acknowledge all the feelings that are present and breathe acceptance of each one. After a few minutes, allow a smile to turn up the corners of your lips. Feel an "inner smile." Begin to breathe in and out of your heart while attuning to something that brings you joy—it could be a child, a beautiful sunset, playing in water, dancing, your pet, or perhaps your partner. Remain there for at least five minutes, or for as long as you like. This can be a beautiful way to return to yourself any time, and also a lovely way to prepare for making love.

☉ Attuning from Outside to Inside

Set aside about half an hour to be on your own without disturbance. Use some music if you like, light a candle, bring a nice fragrance into the room with fresh flowers or pure essences. Lying down, begin with the breath, noticing it coming and going. Not making anything happen. If you feel constricted anywhere, first tighten that part and relax it. Allow your body to soften and widen and be aware this process can take time.

Begin to feel the outside of your skin—what clothing or texture is touching your body. Feel yourself sinking deeper into you. Then imagine you are going a layer deeper than your skin. In other words allow your awareness and your imagination to transport you there. Imagine you are starting to sense yourself from the inside through the layers to the exterior.

As you practice in this way you will start to develop an inner sensitivity to the subtle and fine layers of the body, which will help you become more still in life and lovemaking, more present to yourself. When you develop the art of awakening to your inner experiencing, another world of possibility opens to you. You will notice how it changes your whole being and your whole sense of self.

One female retreat participant told us:

I have always felt a very deep loneliness, but since learning how to be present in my body, I don't feel lonely anymore. With this very simple information I could really get in touch with myself, and actually I found a real "self" inside of me. Now when I relate to others they appear much less "scary" to me, because I am not on my own. It's like my inner child can relax and know everything will be okay. When I put myself in this inner alignment, I find I can take a pause if any energy comes abruptly toward me. I can put a distance between myself and the situation, without swinging this way or that way. And I can feel that I am "not" the situation. Before whenever a situation of stress would arise, it was as if the situation could get a hold of me and overcome me. Also this would happen if it was a situation where I was enthusiastic. And now these days, when any energy comes to me and I am aligned, I can say "this is not me." I am something else. I know that this situation cannot affect my real or true self. Of course it might affect my ego and priorities, but it cannot deeply affect my real self.

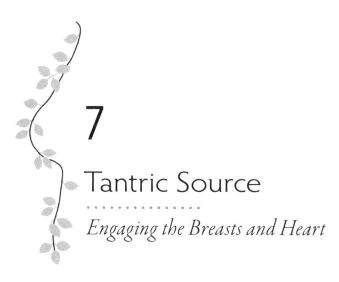

7

Tantric Source

Engaging the Breasts and Heart

FEMALE BREASTS ARE THE ULTIMATE SYMBOL of woman-hood. Breasts have been a source of inspiration for artists and sculptors for thousands of years. They have enchanted and intoxicated, inspired and illuminated. They have been revered for their beautiful curves, soft roundness, the velvety smooth texture of their skin, their pliable shape, and their life-giving potential for feeding babies. In young girls, budding nipples and sprouting pubic hair are usually the first signals of the changes that come with puberty. These changes symbolize the first step into the maiden years, to be followed by adulthood. So delicate can feelings and experiences be at this time that they can have a strong imprint on future feelings about the body, especially in relation to sex.

Some cultures encourage girls to rejoice in their breasts and bodies and celebrate themselves with abandon, whereas most Western cultures imbue young women with a distorted, oversexualized view of their breasts and bodies. It's interesting to note that as sex is spoken about more openly, touted and exposed in media, and widely available visually and otherwise, a whole generation of stoop-shouldered girls has emerged. This posture often indicates feelings of shyness or shame, so perhaps they are attempting to hide their breasts due to the cultural overemphasis on sex.

LACK OF ACCEPTANCE OF BREASTS

Some women feel their breasts are too small and would prefer they be larger. In some urban high schools, girls ask for breast implants as a graduation gift! Other girls who are more "well endowed" try to avoid the attention that large breasts unwittingly attract. One woman remembered that she had felt traumatized by the negative attention she got while growing up and had hated her large breasts ever since. She wasn't ready for the attention being given to a body part she couldn't control. Another young woman may relish her ample gift with great zeal. Again, each woman is so different in her responses. Whatever the situation, women know that breasts gain the attention of men, wanted or otherwise.

As a woman moves through her life, her breasts may be treated in less than loving ways, not least of all by her own self. The cultural trend to pack them neatly into bras with underwire, compressing them against synthetic fabric, indicates we are far more involved in how they look from the outside than how they feel from the inside.

Lovers might also press and hurt them, suck them too hard, or treat them with little awareness at times. Sometimes women have had surgery to remove cysts or have had mastectomies, and some no longer have breasts at all. Some women struggle with breastfeeding, feeling pressured or inadequate about their performance in that regard. Others find that breastfeeding or overstimulation of the nipples has caused a kind of numbness, or a distaste or repulsion toward being touched. There are women who feel embarrassment or shame about their natural breasts. And quite a number of women find that they don't think about their breasts at all and have virtually no awareness within the tissues and flesh. For such women, breasts are of no real consequence at all, except for the outer show.

All in all, few are the women who love their breasts unconditionally, exactly as they are, and yet they are so incredibly significant in both form and function.

BREASTS AS SOURCE

Breasts are understood by Tantra to be the source of a woman's deepest orgasmic experiences. They contain endless potential as a wellspring of sensitivity and ecstatic expansion. These experiences are within every woman's reach when she opens her awareness to the true power of her breasts. Spiritual master Osho recognized this and when he reintroduced the ancient tantric scriptures during the 1970s, he stated that all meditation for women should start at the breasts, as they are the initial source for the rising kundalini energy in a woman's body. Most meditation practices have been invented by men, thus they usually start with the focus at the base of the spine, the source of rising male energy. In women, the breasts and nipples are the female energy-raising pole, the ultimate source of her sexual energy, even for women who have had breasts removed.

It is also possible for a woman to visualize drawing energy from the base (vagina) upward and radiating it out through her breasts, which can have energizing effects. However the vitality in this case is not really being raised from the positive pole, and it is this crucial aspect that is tremendously expansive and deeply transforming. Through a woman melting and merging with her breasts (and thus her heart) she awakens and accesses the true radiance, fragrance, and sweetness of the feminine. This is likely to be a more subtle experience based on sensitivity, rather than an overwhelming or sensational experience.

When a woman tunes in regularly to her breasts she can awaken to the true innate power, sensual vitality, and aliveness available to her. The whole area around the breasts gradually becomes warm, wide, and alive, and the nipples begin to sparkle. These good feelings need to be held in the forefront of her overall awareness of the body. If women wish to open to ecstatic expanded states, whether alone or with a partner, they need to recreate the connection to their breasts and embrace them as the source of female vitality and femininity in a very real way. This is not a goal; rather it is discovering how to open to the breasts in the present moment.

Many women already know to some degree that there is a connection between the breasts and nipples and the vagina through their own sexual experiences. Midwives have known this for eons, that the best way to encourage a laboring woman's cervix to open is to stimulate the nipples or have her husband kiss and fondle them. If we remember that energy in a woman's body is raised via the breasts, and in particular the nipples, and this gives access to the subtle yet vital and beautiful feelings, then we have good reason to cultivate our own love and tenderness for this amazing part of our bodies. We have good reason to love them from the inside rather than focusing on their outward appearance, embracing them as the source, valuing them as an intrinsic gift of the creator.

RECLAIMING THE BREASTS

For the many years up to menopause, you may have felt that your breasts were not yours for pleasure. And if you have breastfed babies, your breasts certainly have not been exclusively yours for a period of time. Many women say they derive an exquisite pleasure from the experience of breastfeeding; a feeling of orgasmic euphoria can arise in a very still and pleasurable way. If you have felt this way, now it's time for you to reclaim them for yourself.

Additionally a woman can easily feel that a man owns her body; often her body has not been for her pleasure, just for a man's (or men's) pleasure. The conditioning to please and make man happy is so powerful, and a woman's fear of losing her man is so deep, that she may have allowed her body to be touched and treated in ways that do not please her.

For sure, when a woman gets a true yes with the feeling of willingness coursing through her body, all she may want to do is to offer her breasts to her beloved, in all their fullness and glory. All too easily though, if the bodily yes is not forthcoming, a woman gives up and gives in to him, forgetting about and overriding herself. Some things might have felt a bit off, too difficult, too fast perhaps, a bit insensitive, but she goes ahead anyway. This can lead to various emotional consequences including rage, anger, and sadness, or a sense of disconnection or separation.

Meditate on Your Breasts Daily

To cultivate your female energy we suggest that you meditate on your breasts daily, as outlined later in this chapter. For ten to twenty minutes, when you wake up and when you go to sleep, just holding them gently is a wonderful way to bring this feminine quality into your life. Simply remembering to bring awareness to your breasts at any time during the day will support you in making it a practice of entering the body *through* your positive energy-raising pole. You can tune in to your breasts while you are working on your computer, while preparing a meal, or while chatting with a friend, for example. It's as simple as, once again, inverting our attention inward, sensing both breasts from the inside equally, and feeling as if the nipples are radiating energy outward. You can use visualization as a support. Be aware that it may take quite some time and practice to begin to perceive the subtle tingling, swelling, and almost imperceptible energy being activated.

If you notice aliveness in the corresponding negative or receptive pole, the vagina and womb, it indicates that you are tuned in to the inner rod of magnetism described in chapter 3. Some women find when they first try this that they don't feel anything, or feel very little. Keep going; it actually happens anyway. It's just that you have not been aware of it up until now. It may take days, weeks, or months. A sixty-years-young woman reported that it took her six weeks of daily practice before she could begin to feel this inner vitality. Some women may need longer. The experience is a subtle, fine, delicate one, not an overwhelming or intense one, yet this is the doorway to inner feminine radiance. A grace and presence exudes from the woman who is in touch with her femininity on this level. You quite naturally arrive "home" when you begin to contact the power of the breasts and use them in your best interests.

As we know, the breasts frame the heart area, both energetically and physically, as the center of love. So when you do make breast meditation and breast awareness part of your daily practice, love seems to naturally radiate from you.

As you start to feel the breasts from the inside and practice connecting with them, you then have a place to share from when you make love with your partner. There is empowerment in claiming them for yourself and a feeling of energetic expansion that seems to magnetize others to you, especially your partner. In lovemaking, love exudes from the woman who is in touch with her inner vitality and she may find a man enters quite effortlessly and naturally into her space. A sweet, unapologetic self-confidence rises for a woman who is willing to open herself to these subtle divine energies.

Removal of Breasts

It is extremely important for women to know that the energy-raising pole still exists even in the absence of a physical breast, so this is some encouragement in challenging circumstances. When women who have had breast removal meditate on their breasts and "feel" their nipples where they would have been, they find that they can contact the energy and also feel its corresponding flow to the vagina. It requires placing awareness inside and visualizing the breasts. Energy flows where awareness goes.

Diana says,

In my earliest years of teaching, I remember a woman who'd had cancer and a double mastectomy fourteen years prior. She discovered that through placing her awareness on her breasts energetically from the inside, she was able to feel a resonance in the vagina and for the first time since her surgery had natural lubrication. Her story made it clear that the absence of physical breasts did not interfere with the deep-seated magnetic polarity. This intrinsic response in the body has since been confirmed by several other women in the same situation.

The following is a true story of Janet's experience with the breast meditation.

THE ZURICH STORY

I was in Zurich a few years ago and found myself with half an hour to wait to meet my partner outside our hotel. The hotel was by the river Limmat, and outside were lovely little tables right on the river where the Swiss enjoy their coffees and other drinks.

Instead, though, I decided to go back up to my room and use the time to lie on the bed and relax, and the way I relax these days is to do what is called a "breast meditation," which I learned through Diana.

It's easy. I just lie down and imagine melting into my breasts, relaxing and sensing them from the inside, and bringing awareness to the heart area. Sometimes I may feel a streaming of energy that is fine and subtle, and flows down into the womb and vagina.

I lay there for half an hour, not forcing anything, just relaxing, relaxing. Then I got up, fixed my hair, and went down to the lobby and outside. What happened in the next few minutes was like something out of a movie! Honestly, it was incredible. It was like I was experiencing each moment frame by frame.

The second I walked into the lobby a man in his forties met my eye and smiled. As he passed and I moved forward, all the men behind the front desk looked up. I walked through the turnstile and was greeted by the concierge. Well, that always happens. . . . Then I looked to my left and about twelve men were waiting on the corner in a huddle; most of them turned and met my eyes. I walked further into the courtyard looking around for my partner, who had not yet appeared. Right in front of me was a man in his thirties leaning against a car with two women. He sat up and his face lit up as he smiled and greeted me. Of course I smiled back and said hello. Wondering at this stage what the hell was going on, I kind of smiled inside—well, I'm human . . .

it's nice to be over fifty and still get a little attention. Then I turned back toward the hotel and went to the right where the high-set coffee tables were by the river. As I brushed past another man in his late fifties, he greeted me, too! I smiled, said hi, and moved on. My goodness! What was going on? I've never had men I don't even know speaking to me like that in just a few moments. I've had them look but not approach me and actually say something. And then again! Another man moved toward me and greeted me—all very respectfully, no weird stuff going on. By this time I was really smiling and thinking this bloody breast meditation stuff really works! My Swiss friend Nathalie was so surprised when I told her this; she said Swiss men never speak to women like that. And all this happened, frame by frame, in literally the space of about two minutes. It has really convinced me of the subtle power that a woman has for drawing the masculine presence toward her. I was not trying to make anything happen, just innocently looking around for my friend. I believe it was not how I looked physically—I was not wearing high heels or a short skirt, or revealing my breasts, none of the usual trademark looks to get attention.

Women become irresistible and appealing to men when they rest in their own natural feminine presence. This is not something that one woman can have and not others; this is the equal force that every woman innately has, irrespective of age or appearance, and has the potential to experience.

No Goals

It's crucial to enter into the breast meditation without wanting to get any result, not making any kind of goal out of it. When I (Janet) did this meditation in my hotel room, it was not to get something, it was simply to just be, and to relax within my body. There were no fireworks, no huge sensational experience, no techniques, or even moving the body— no focusing on anything, just being, just melting, relaxing, being, in my own body. I noticed that subtle feelings of joy would arise in me as a result of doing this.

So don't try so hard! For both single women and women in partnerships, if you are wanting to feel more attuned to yourself and wish to feel more confident with a man, just relax more, soften into yourself, be more present in your body, feel yourself instead of attempting to make interesting conversation or pretending to be something that you're not. And experiment with the breast meditation later in this chapter. Also keep in mind this is not a goal or strategy to attract a man, but rather a way to experience the complete beauty of the inner sensual nature of your own female body.

Increasing Feeling in the Breasts

Naturally breasts connect with the heart area and thus with love; there are no errors in nature. Many women ask, because they find it difficult to connect with the breasts inwardly, if they can instead just tune in to the heart for awakening their female energy. Yes, this is also possible, but the fact is that the breasts and nipples are the key to awakening and accessing the special biomagnetic circulation in the female body, and not the heart center per se. Ultimately, however, when the breasts open in this way, it also opens the heart.

To also increase sensitivity in the breasts, try to locate a sometimes very sensitive spot right between the breasts, on the breastbone, and in line with where the nipples would have been as a young girl. That is a helpful place to massage lightly. Use the fingertips of one hand and make a circular motion. Sometimes the place can feel a bit tense and oversensitive but this should change after a bit of massage. You can also include the entire surface of the sternum/breastbone, lightly massaging the area with small circular movements, as well as each of the intercostal spaces (spaces between the ribs) where the ribs connect with the breastbone. This central chest area can have a very significant effect on arousal when touched, feathered, or kissed sensitively. In fact, any area of the décolletage can be a highly sensitive area when touched lightly. Experimenting with your own body is a beautiful way to be in touch with this exquisite part of you.

Breast Augmentation

The number of women having breast implants has nearly tripled since 1997,* with the majority of women having the procedure in their twenties, thirties, and forties, some in their teens. This indicates that more and more women moving into their menopause years will have had breast surgery. Whether it be for cosmetic, health, or other reasons, this is a personal choice. It's interesting to note that breast sensitivity is definitely affected by breast implants. Some indicate it lessens sensitivity between 40 to 60 percent. Certainly women who have been in our retreats have reported that it is not so easy to feel their nipples and breasts while doing the breast meditation. We believe that with practice and awareness it is possible that some meaningful level of sensitivity can be cultivated.

Old Feelings May Move On

The whole chest region, however (and it is the same for a man), can also be where a woman becomes guarded energetically, and due to past painful experiences it is almost like she is wearing a chest plate. So there is an unconscious armoring or protection or defensive pattern there, which limits feeling in the tissues. At times you may even sense an ache, or a kind of protective barrier over that whole region. This is where we can easily unconsciously brace, contract, and become a bit cut off and a bit disconnected if we have not softened and allowed some shedding of these old protective layers.

With the reawakening of this area of the breasts, a woman might find in the process of lovemaking or during meditation that something of her past dislodges and tears may flow to the release these protective layers that constrict the heart from loving and being open to love. These layers, if not attended to, may make loving and sustaining love more difficult. It's good to approach these feelings with tenderness and compassion. There will be more discussion of this aspect and how to manage it in chapter 10.

---

*Source: http://www.ourbodiesourselves.org/health-info/facts-about-breast-implants.

HEART REJUVENATION

The heart has its own intelligence. It is said that simply breathing in and out of the heart area, associating pleasant thoughts and feelings with the breath, increases DHEA, the youth and health hormone, by 100 percent over a few weeks, as mentioned in chapter 2. Remember this decreases the stress hormone cortisol, thus nourishing the adrenal glands, which virtually every perimenopausal and menopausal woman needs.

We always notice how women are looking ten to twenty years younger by the end of the Making Love Retreats—only seven days! In fact, within three days the first signs of rejuvenation are clearly visible. This regeneration is the by-product of body awareness, containment, and inner expansion, rather than contraction and dispersal of energy. Revival happens when relaxation replaces tension, which in turn creates the possibility of allowing love in, of receiving it, and also letting love flow, of sharing it. When a woman is relaxed she is spontaneously more loving. You may have noticed when you go on vacation you are more likely to want to make love; you feel more present and open without the stresses of everyday life.

⏥ Loving Your Own Breasts

Take the time on your own, away from everyone else, and give yourself the space to touch your own breasts. Make some space for yourself for twenty to thirty minutes. Soften the lighting in your room or use candles. Play your favorite relaxing music. Prepare a fragrance using your favorite essential oils. Rose oil is the fragrance of love and is beautiful for the breasts. Avoid citrus oils as they tend to burn. Set yourself up with sarongs and towels to avoid spillage. Warming the oil first is lovely, or just warm it in your hands. You can be seated or lying down.

Gently oil the breasts, molding and gently massaging them with upward or circular movements. Stroke and caress them, feel them, feather them, look at them, and without labeling them as good or bad, simply feel their soft or even scarred texture. Allow whatever feelings present themselves to gently arise. Open to these feelings and welcome them, inviting them back into your life if you have been estranged from them. It can be very powerful and healing to allow these old stored feelings to rise to the surface and be released.

It also can be soothing to sit in the sunlight and feel your naked breasts and nipples being warmed by the heat of the sun, of course being careful not to burn the delicate skin, just for ten minutes or so. With each breath imagine that you are sipping light in and out of the nipples.

⊙ Breast Meditation

Including the breast meditation in your life is an act of self-love. It entitles you to open to yourself before you open to another. Sexual energy is transformed into love through simple awareness of the visceral, somatic experiencing of the body. When you practice entering the awareness of the body and tuning in to subtle feelings and finer movements of energy residing within your body, the self can melt into love without effort. Things that seemed important an hour ago become insignificant and you start to comprehend that the only truly significant thing is love. When you experience yourself as the source of love, you will feel the cells of your body vibrating as pure love.

This meditation is best done on a bed or long sofa where you can comfortably stretch out, lying on your back, legs straight and parallel. Place a pillow or a blanket rolled into a long sausage shape under the knees, so that the knees are slightly curved, releasing pressure on the lower back and helping the legs to relax. Place a pillow under the neck and head, but not too high, more flat, and be sure that the neck and head form one line in relation to the spine and lower body. This very precise body alignment, described at the end of chapter 3, will enable you to gain more access to your inner body and make it easier for you to be present.

Close your eyes. Relax and breathe. Tune in by bringing your awareness into your breasts and nipples, sensing into them without any direct touch. If it helps to get a sense of the nipples, you can brush them lightly three or four times. After several minutes, cup each breast with your hands, one each, lifting up from the side of the ribcage, inward and upward, so that the nipples are more or less at their "original" position, if possible. The breasts are floating in your hands, not being squashed or compressed by them. Start to become aware of and relax tensions you notice in your body, and then begin sensing and being with your breasts from within for about twenty to thirty minutes.

It's not a strong focus or concentration, more of a melting and merging, a dissolving into them. And at some point during this time frame, it is highly possible that you will suddenly snap back to normal reality, returning feeling refreshed, energized, and uplifted. Lie still for a few minutes or for as long as you wish, then slowly roll onto your side and come to a sitting position.

Some women report that the elbows get uncomfortable after holding the cupping position for a while. If that is your experience, try next time with pillows under the elbows to support them, and if that does not help, simply straighten the arms and let them lie at your side, palms facing upward. Some women prefer not to touch their breasts at all and find it disturbing, which is also fine. The main objective is to feel the breasts from the inside; the hands are only a support to draw the awareness into them. The significant aspect is developing the capacity to feel this area from within, to contact it on a fine, sweet, subtle cellular level.

Remember developing sensitivity takes time and practice. Go in with innocence and openness, no expectations, with the intention to be present in the body and see what is revealed to you through this new orientation. Like a traveler you have a map, but the territory looks quite different and your quest is to traverse that very territory with an adventurous and intrepid spirit, enjoying the journey in its unfolding flow.

LOOKING AFTER YOUR BREASTS—
THE FEMALE LYMPH SYSTEM

The breast meditation is a beautiful way to bring your breasts into your awareness and to be more conscious of them. Your body will be grateful for any loving attention you give it. Another loving way to care for your breasts is to gently massage the lymphatic system. This is very important for breast health, activates lymphatic drainage, increases blood flow, and gently activates the tissues. If you are in touch with your breasts on a regular basis, you will be able to detect any change in the tissue. The following lymphatic massage comes from Dr. Christiane Northrup.* The self-massage technique was developed by Dana Wyrick, who practices lymphedema therapy at Mesa Physical Therapy/San Diego Virtual Lymphedema Clinic in San Diego, California.

⌷ Self-Massage of Lymph System near Chest and Breasts

Work on each side of your chest independently. Instructions below are for the left side. Simply reverse hand instructions when you're ready to address your right side. Use a light touch. Your object is to move the skin, not to massage the muscles. The following routine, when done properly, will assist the lymphatic capillaries in removing toxins and impurities from body tissue. The stroking will also accelerate transport of impurities to the lymph nodes where they will be processed and rendered harmless. Finally, cleansed lymph will be returned to the bloodstream where the now harmless impurities may be carried to the lung, kidneys, and colon for elimination.

1. With the first three fingers of your right hand, locate the hollow above your left collarbone. Stroking from your shoulders toward your neck, lightly stretch your skin in the hollow. Repeat this movement five to ten times.
2. Now cover the hair-growth part of your left armpit with the fingers of your right hand held very flat. Stretch the skin of your armpit upward five to ten times.

---

*Christiane Northrup, M.D., *The Wisdom of Menopause: Creating Physical and Emotional Health during the Change* (New York: Bantam Books, 2012), 538.

3. Again using a flat right hand, lightly stroke (pet) the skin from the breastbone to the armpit. Do this above the breast, over the breast and below the breast, repeating each path five to ten times.

4. Finally, using a flat right hand, lightly stroke from your left wrist up to your left armpit along the inner arm, repeating five to ten times.

Now change hands and attend to the right side of your chest following the same sequence with your left hand.

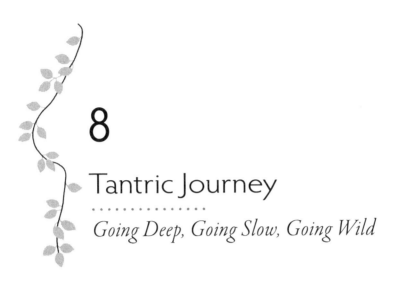

8

Tantric Journey

Going Deep, Going Slow, Going Wild

MANY PERIMENOPAUSAL AND MENOPAUSAL WOMEN report feeling such a lack of desire for sex that they feel totally disheartened. They are concerned that they are not living up to the image of what a sexy, alive woman should look like, that it's an image they can't relate to. However, such views only hold true as long as we see ourselves from the outside and in an external way. Reclaiming your body and becoming increasingly "embodied" implies seeing, feeling, and experiencing yourself from the inside, rather than continually referencing yourself from the outside.

LACK OF DESIRE AS SPIRITUAL GATEWAY

Menopause clears the pathway from the emphasis on sexual desire, because for more than half of women at this time, desire seems to no longer be there. It asks us, then, to go deeper, to look deeper, to feel more deeply. The body often won't take fast and unconscious anymore, won't take mechanical friction anymore, won't take what has been before, which, if a woman is curious enough, clears and opens an alternative path that is more restful for the menopausal woman and her lover. Many think there is no way in sex anymore, that something is wrong with them, and that's where women become disheartened and give up on their marriage, relationship, or their own sex life.

This is fact: around 75 percent of women's bodies (and not only menopausal women) can no longer tolerate the mechanical vaginal friction of conventional sex without consequences of pain, discontent, or closure (www.theothered.com). But this also suggests a gateway, a gift, a shift. Menopause begs a woman's body to become more tantric, relaxed, and present. It invites her to go deeper and slower in her whole life, to be free and, in fact, more "wild," as in more authentic, more natural, and a more honest expression of her true essence. Despite a lack of classic desire, women who step over that threshold and follow the guidelines we have given will find that they have no trouble eventually feeling sexually interested. They might also move into an expanded orgasmic state, which is very different from a peak orgasm.

Wild Is Pure Presence

Almost like a primitive call from the wild, another way emerges. It challenges the female conditioning that dictates pleasing a man, being immediately ready, and fulfilling his every desire. Making love in relaxation and awareness, particularly with awareness on your breasts, connects you to this call from the wild inner self, where you must deeply listen to your own body and psyche, and trust its call and timing. If you think of the characteristics of a wild animal, "wild" is pure presence, spontaneous, natural, and instinctive, but not out of control, unconscious, or sensation seeking.

Wild is sensitive, aware of its surroundings. It has composure. Wild moves the body on impulse, in the moment without preconceived thought. Wild rests when rest arrives. Wild is naturally playful. It's this level of truly open, unbridled wildness you can bring to your lovemaking. Wildness in the conventional sense may imply getting out of control with heat and passion, expelling the energy with a climactic peak, but the wildness we refer to here is much softer, simpler, and more relaxing. Think of the splendor of a lioness lazing in the sun.

As Diana wrote in an earlier book, "As far as wildness is concerned, it's a matter for redefinition. What we know as wild in sex is usually pretty unconscious, lust driven, tense, and mechanical. So in this sense the experience is desensitizing, because there is a tendency to contract at a deep level and there will be little room for expansion. As I understand and experience it, lust and passion are two different states. Lust has a direction, a buildup, some climax. Passion, on the other hand, is pure presence, going nowhere, relaxed, senses totally open, nothing forced. True wildness is at one with nature, utterly sensitive and conscious, opening to the moment through the body. Wildness has no pattern; the bodies spontaneously flow and form amazing configurations."*

Passionately Undemonstrative

Australian spiritual teacher Barry Long recommends that a woman be "passionately undemonstrative." These two words seem to oppose each other, yet if you contemplate them you can start to get a feel for their incredible meaning. It does not mean passive or inactive in lovemaking; it is more about each person being totally present and not "doing" anything special other than being fully anchored in her or his own body. The woman is not moving outward with her attention, but poised with resting awareness. This makes her available, receptive, and spontaneous.

This body connection makes her powerfully passionate in a very unconventional sense of the word. She is pure presence itself—pure passion. She is vital yet stillness resides in her being. The passion is not outward going, directed on someone else or on releasing energy; rather it is contained and transforms into a rising vital and revitalizing force. Passion is pure presence. The by-product of being passionately undemonstrative allows the life force to move through her. The by-product of being outwardly demonstrative is usually excitement and a dispersing of energy. There is nothing wrong with that, but if she wants to

*Diana Richardson, *Tantric Love Letters: A Collection of Experiences, Questions, and Answers* (Arlesford, Hants, U.K.: "O" Books, 2011), 155.

recalibrate her sexual experience into love, and to harness the aliveness and depth of her femininity, then contemplating the meaning of these words, and practicing with them, is a worthwhile adventure.

Returning Intelligence to Our Genitals

In lovemaking the way forward is that you actually let the bodies lead the way, following their more natural flow and allowing the organs themselves to guide you. Giving space to the organs to "do their own complementary thing" in an environment of serenity and peace returns intelligence to the genitals. This level of innate intelligence is absolutely unheard of in conventional sex.

To shift our experience we must invite an even deeper level of presence and let go of ideas about orgasm or ejaculation/peak experiences. As already mentioned, being more conscious in our movement, our breath, our touch will naturally result in more slowness, heightening our senses, and allowing spaciousness for love to flow more freely.

The healing potential and power of an organic intimate connection between man and woman can grow exponentially as each becomes increasingly present to every moment of making love, and the ensuing slowness and delicious qualities of orgasmic expansion remain in the body for a long time after having sex. We have repeatedly heard women say that they feel like everything got put back together again after lovemaking in this way. It settles the being on a profound level that really compares to nothing else. There is a sense of being in alignment and in complete harmony.

Soft Entry

With less excitement and stimulation, erections may not happen readily. Another totally viable alternative is "soft entry," placing the penis into the vagina while it is relaxed. This is a beautiful way to begin sex and encourages staying in that cooler zone. It enables you both to start at the same place, where a man's sexual temperature is more in the resting zone rather than already in the heated phase. If you feel you just want to simply connect, even if you don't feel you have much interest or energy for sex, then the option of relaxed or soft entry can be a wonderful, no-pressure way to be together—just resting, like a meditation.

If you have a history of pain or thinning walls of the vagina, as can happen during menopause or earlier, this simple way of connecting the genitals helps enormously. If pain or thinning is the case, it's always good to start with the penis resting *only* at the entrance of the vagina, while bringing awareness and melting into your breasts. Meanwhile, the man similarly brings his awareness to the base of his penis—the perineum area. The side scissors position, as shown in figure 8.1 on page 112, is optimal for soft entry. Man lies on his side and woman lies on her back as they intertwine their legs and bring the genital areas together. You can always use pillows to prop under legs or hips, depending on body shapes. It's helpful if you first spread your labia a bit with your hands and place the penis, flesh to flesh, resting gently at the opening of the vagina.

This is a lovely way to start making love. Typically, man wants to get inside woman as soon as he can because of the fear of losing his erection. But if the woman encourages him to relax, they both might find that after allowing the first erection to go down, and being together in this relaxed way, erection is very likely to return. It can even be beneficial, as sometimes the first erection may be a little charged, the penis very hard and excited, and entering in this more neutral way allays the situation where the man might gallop ahead of the woman. The second and subsequent erections are likely to be less tense and less driven by excitement, with the penis firm yet supple and pliable.

There is a great misconception that if a man is not erect then he has little male potency. Men are often surprised to find that a woman is usually able to literally feel the flow of the dynamic force when a penis is resting inside her vagina, even if it is not erect. Starting with soft entry creates the opportunity for the vagina to receive a relaxed penis, which softens the tissues and enables the vagina to open and widen with ease. Lubrication with natural oils is a great support. Coconut, walnut, and pomegranate oils are highly recommended.

The soft entry alternative is a welcome opportunity for a woman who has some thinning of the vaginal walls and faces pain and discomfort whenever a hard, erect penis pushes into the vagina. The simplicity of the start enables a woman to relax into her being and body and tune in to herself, rather than brace for pain.

Position for Soft Entry

Importantly, soft entry takes the pressure off the man by disproving the assumption that the penis must be erect in order to make love. So if a man is having difficulties with erection in the absence of direct stimulation, or if he experiences impotence, soft entry means he can still connect with a woman and make love to her. When the penis is inserted in its relaxed state, the man is given the opportunity to be more present, since the pressure of *having to have* an erection can often lead to psychological distress or sexual fantasy. With relaxed entry this pitfall is eliminated. Managing to insert the relaxed penis in the vagina is a knack that takes some practice, but it is well worth it.

A male retreat participant shares the following feedback on soft entry:

I had stopped approaching my wife for sex as it was always too painful for her and the last thing I want to do is hurt her. After trying out soft entry, we have now found a way to unite and share love in a simple relaxing way, without pain for her, and that has been a life changer for us and our relationship.

And a female retreat participant had this to say:

Soft entry really works for me because I can relax more without pressure, and I was amazed to discover that I can feel the delicate energies emanating from my man's penis even though it's not erect. In fact it was more deeply satisfying and touching.

The position for soft entry is relatively easy and is sometimes called the scissors position. As shown in figure 8.1, the man lies on his side with a pillow under his head and faces the woman. The woman lies on her back, bringing her pelvis close to his. Both open their legs and the genitals will be naturally lying opposite each other. Bring the genitals together and also intertwine your legs and fit into each other—in scissor-like fashion—as shown in the figure below. Note that the bottom leg should always be the man's, and the top leg should always be the woman's. The woman may need to move her upper body away from her lover's so that she is at almost a 90-degree angle to him in order to make the pelvises fit together nicely. Or she can angle her own pelvis upward. Experiment to find out what is most comfortable. This position does not work for every couple right away but it is worth trying several times without giving up immediately if you don't get it on the first try. The figure shows the man lying to the left of his partner, but it is advisable to change sides from time to time, with woman on the left and man on the right.

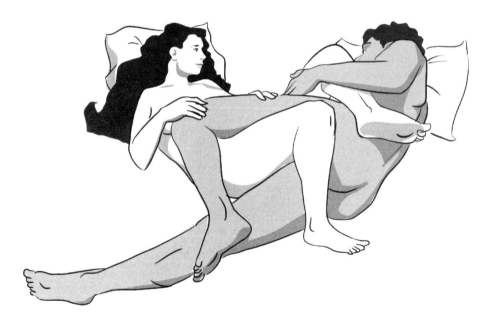

Fig. 8.1. Side position suitable for soft entry

Woman Inserts the Penis

Once you are positioned correctly and comfortably, with pelvises close together and the vagina opposite the penis, then woman can proceed to guide the penis inside her. If you need lubricant (highly advisable), now would be the perfect moment to apply it liberally on all the relevant surfaces. First spread lubricant at your vaginal entrance and then on the labia. After that spread the labia wide apart, using one hand on each side, and expose the vaginal entrance. Then spread oil on the head and shaft of the penis, but avoid an excess of oil so that the penis doesn't get too slippery to handle. Then take the penis in your hands and gently pull or roll back any folds of foreskin or tissue around the head of the penis, thus exposing the penis head.

As shown in figure 8.2, you now make a two-pronged fork with the first two fingers of both hands (short fingernails are important so the woman does not scratch her vagina). Place one finger fork (try the left hand) firmly around the base of the penis and hold it there. With the other hand (the right) place the first two fingers directly behind and to

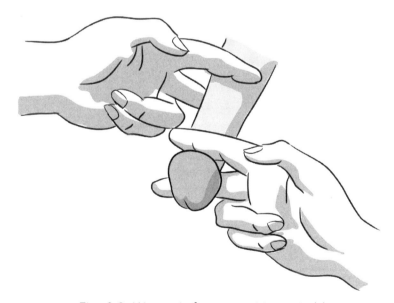

Fig. 8.2. Woman's finger position suitable
for managing soft entry

either side of the rim that encircles the head of the penis. Squeeze the fingers together so that you have a gentle grip on the penis, and then pull the penis toward your vagina. When it arrives at the entrance begin to insert it. You will be able to push the penis in and up a little way. Move the fingers back a little bit, and then again grip the penis between your two fingers and direct it into your vagina.

By repeating the finger movement again and again, it is as if you're feeding or walking the penis into the vagina, pushing him inside a little more each time. Once you have got all of it inside you (or as much as you can manage to insert—even to get the head in is a good start), remove your hands and bring the pelvic areas together as close as possible, then intertwine your legs around each other and relax! Use pillows to make yourselves as comfortable as you can, and use previously given suggestions that support your presence. In this side position eye contact is easy and important, as is breathing, and it is possible too for the man to rest a hand/s on the woman's breast/s while the woman in turn can stroke and caress his pelvis and legs.

Relax Belly when Inserting Penis

You absolutely must keep your vagina relaxed when you get to the point of actually inserting the penis, or it will be like trying to force your lover through a closed door—it simply won't work. Naturally as you get ready, you will want to look between your legs to see what you are doing, especially at first. You will do this by contracting the belly musculature and lifting your upper body. However when the belly contracts, so does the vagina, so to avoid this inevitable tightening and narrowing of the vagina, which will make getting the penis into you more difficult, lie back on the mattress for a few moments to relax and widen the vagina. Do this once you have hold of the penis *and before insertion,* and you will be able to get the penis inside more easily. So always remember to lie back first, then send your awareness downward into the vagina, keeping it relaxed and open, and then slip the penis in. The more you practice, the easier it gets. You can use soft entry as a very viable option for approaching lovemaking every time if you wish, or use it when you need it. The scissors position is a relaxing start for soft entry but any time you feel that you need to move, you can change position.

A NEW SEXUAL LANGUAGE

As you embark on a new and more relaxed way of uniting, it is so helpful to communicate what you are feeling. For instance, when a man hears from his partner that she can feel energy radiating from his soft, non-erect penis, that is a great relief. Discovering that he is alive when he's soft is extremely reassuring. He can stop worrying about erection and focus his attention on the direct experience of the penis within the vagina. This is a far more subtle level of perception and requires a quietness of mind and absence of anxious thoughts.

Bringing the bodies together in this way opens up all kinds of other possibilities for sexual exchange. Just leave it up to the genitals supported by your consciousness, and they will do whatever feels right to them. It is a completely new sexual language. The penis may lie in the vagina, humming quietly and contentedly, or after a while it may start vibrating strongly. It may become slowly and steadily erect, pushing high up into the vagina, dancing and jerking upward, or relax down again, snaking all the way out, only to rise back up again in thrilling penetration. Through this meeting of opposites, all kinds of miracles happen.

A woman can still become pregnant while in perimenopause, so if you are using a condom, it's important to do so only with a pharmaceutical lubricant, such as K-Y Jelly, or preferably, and more highly recommended for the health of your vagina, a more natural water-based lubricant such as organic Good Clean Love. *Absolutely do not lubricate with oil* while using a condom as it will disintegrate the rubber and cause the condom to provide no protection. Suitable oils for lubrication when not using a condom are coconut, walnut, sesame, or pomegranate. All oils and lubricants should be without perfume or scent. Coconut has a beautiful consistency for lovemaking. It can be inserted into the vagina where it instantly melts, creating a silky smooth effect.

Marlene had been experiencing severe sexual pain and shared how relieved she was to discover a new way of making love:

Here is a short report about my sexual history in this lifetime. First let me thank you with all my heart for this wonderful love retreat, which created a total turning point in my sexual life. I would never have believed it had I not experienced it myself. After thirty-six years of a loving marriage, yet without any real sexual intercourse, my husband died. A few years later I came across your article about slow sex in an esoteric journal. I wondered: What is slow sex? *Curious enough, I bought your* Slow Sex *DVD,* wherein couples speak about their sexual experiences and especially about the big relief of not necessarily having to manage or achieve an orgasm each time they have sex. What a relief for men and women!*

Shortly after that I met my actual partner and had, of course, similar problems with him: tightness, fear, pain, feeling of culpability, and shyness about how and what to do. I decided to invite him to your Making Love Retreat. Several times he told me it would not work if we did not practice regularly before going there, but I simply could not manage to, it was too painful. Finally we arrived at the retreat and he mentioned our problem and how much effort it is on his side to enter my vagina.

You told us then to start very, very slowly, with vegetable oil, trying to enter softly and slowly, just a little bit, not forcing anything. We tried it out the same day and . . . it worked, to my utter surprise! The position was the one where both are lying on their sides. I was able, by myself, to put his penis head inside me, just a little bit, and there was no pain. Before, it was always very difficult and very painful for me, every movement, maybe because I was too stressed. So we continued and every day it went better and deeper and I started to trust and to let go of my fear. One of the main reasons for my relaxing was that we both knew

---

*Diana Richardson, *Slow Sex: How Sex Makes You Happy—A New Style of Loving*, DVD, 80 minutes (Cologne, Germany: Innenvelt Verlag, 2011).

there was no peak, no orgasm, no special excitement necessary to be performed. Just let him enter softly and "just be"!

At one point, some days into the retreat, I had an insight. I saw that the penis is a flow of love that enters my vagina, which is equally an instrument, a container, and a vessel of love, and that both come together to merge in love. After that it became very easy for me to open my vagina, to let him enter into me and feel oneness. I am seventy years old and my partner is sixty-six years old. Never would I have imagined such a miracle. It is absolute happiness, totally natural, and a feeling of being "one." Thank you for this wonderful help. I wish you a very blessed time and that you continue to help people like me, who had almost no more hope.

Marlene contacted us again, eighteen months later:

My partner and I are still in positive continuation of the practice after two retreats now, and the definite secret is what we were told the first day at our first seminar—not to force the entering of the penis into the vagina but just enter slightly, a little bit and then take a rest, and give the vagina time to relax and open herself, without any forcing, so the relaxation can take place and finally the penis enters slowly and naturally, without any pain. Without this step we would not have succeeded because it was too painful for me, but now it is smooth, pleasant, and we call it the divine union, oneness in the yin and yang, female and male. It's like a miracle, really.

THE CLITORIS DEBATE

There is no doubt that stimulation of the clitoris provides a woman with great pleasure. For women who struggle to orgasm in conventional sex through the vagina, and many do, the clitoris can be a welcome alternative, as it is the easiest way to orgasm. There are said to be eight thousand nerve endings in the clitoris alone, double that of a man's penis. And in fact, interestingly, it grows in size as a woman reaches menopause—up to 2.5 times longer than the clitoris of a pubescent girl.

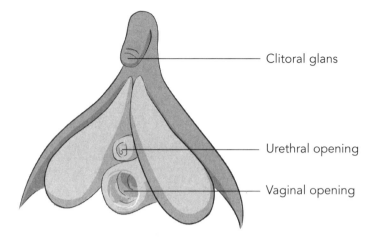

Fig. 8.3. Diagram of clitoris showing urethra
and vaginal openings*

From conception until twelve weeks, all fetal genital tissue is the same. After twelve weeks it begins to differentiate into either a penis or labia. The clitoris swells when aroused and even has a foreskin, a "hood," and a tiny shaft. When looked at anatomically it looks much like a tiny penis. In a way it's surprising as it could be said that it has similar properties to the penis. If the clitoris is masturbated too often or addressed with repeated light stimulating friction, the result is likely to be a fast peak and downward release of energy and with that an ensuing lack of sensitivity and a desire to raise the level of stimulation.

Stimulation of the Clitoris and Its Effects

Repeated overstimulation of the clitoris as a general strategy can have ultimately desensitizing side effects on the vagina, similar in effect to fast, hot, mechanical sex with rapid and forced movement. If you really take the time to observe how you feel afterward, you may notice that you are not so much at peace but feel/sense an agitated emotional residue in the body. When women have heard how constant stimulation of the clitoris can affect them in an adverse way, and start to take

*Source: https://en.wikipedia.org/wiki/Clitoris.

note of this aspect in themselves, they also report these same "negative" outcomes. Some women report a sense of numbness and a kind of deadening of the sexual energy. At times a woman can feel not only emotionally disturbed but also distracted and tense, not at all fulfilled.

The clitoris, in view of its many nerve endings, would perhaps welcome a more sensitive and conscious entry into the beautiful vagina, where the clitoral tissues are not being compressed. When pressure occurs it can inhibit a woman's sexual response. The tension that is usually applied to create the sensation necessary for orgasm via clitoral stimulation accumulates and remains in the system, and in the very organs themselves. The distance between clitoris and vagina varies from woman to woman. In some they are closer together, so in conventional sex, stimulation through penis movement happens more easily; some are further apart, therefore not so easily stimulated by the penis.

The Garden of Love

Invariably fascination with the clitoris directs the focus of both parties to the *outside* of her body, bypassing the connection with the natural wilder intelligence of her vagina and its deeper layers, especially the upper reaches of the vagina around the cervix, the entrance to the womb. We refer to this noteworthy area around the cervix as the "garden of love." If we wish to move in the direction of expansion and more elevated experiences, rather than contraction and release, then it helps to approach the clitoris with less vigor and more sensitivity, or even leave her alone. This is contrary advice, undoubtedly, but its wisdom can be experienced personally by trying it. Basically it is relatively easy for most women to reach orgasm through clitoral stimulation. However the clitoris is not the vagina, the receptor of male energy, so it's good to experiment with not directly stimulating the clitoris in the beginning, rather leave it until much later on, or only occasionally, rather than regularly.

As already mentioned, clitoral stimulation can leave a woman feeling a bit ungrounded, tense, or disconnected. But most importantly, stimulation of the clitoris creates excitement and fills the vaginal tissues with a kind of hunger, or demand, so what is actually happening on a magnetic level is that the intrinsically receptive absorbing organ is turning into an overcharged and agitated area. That will change the whole direction of the lovemaking because the penis reacts to this excitement and so sex is likely to be hotter and more climax oriented.

Vagina Wide and Relaxed

The intention of the woman is to create a receptive and serene environment within the vagina, so that when the penis enters, the man has the sense of being invited and welcomed. That quality of engagement will establish the whole tone of the lovemaking, with a higher level of presence for both. The more relaxed, receptive, and present (passionately undemonstrative) a woman is able to be, the more she has the capacity to draw the man into her reality and exert a "force" that has an impact on his body and being. By paying attention to energetic correspondence between the vagina and penis in this way, a woman can have a lot more influence on the sex act than she may have realized. She can cultivate and nurture her receptive qualities through breast awareness and honoring the entrance of her vagina as a sacred doorway to her garden of love—an entrance to protect, revere, and preserve.

Going In, Staying In
(Deep Sustained Penetration)

Many women know the feeling of being penetrated deep on the inside, where her lover has "kissed" her garden of love with the head of his penis, and how deeply satisfying and profoundly blissful it can feel. It is here in the deeper upper reaches of the vagina that the wild, unique natural fragrance of femininity can flood through her and her lover. When she is touched here by the highly sensitive magnetic head of the penis, and she remains passionately undemonstrative without giving sex direction, profound bliss and deep healing is available. The whole aspect of healing is elaborated in the next chapter.

When a woman allows a man to enter this tender territory without friction and heat, there is an opening of the body, heart, and psyche. Some women cry. Some feel they are opening to the Divine. It will be different every time. As you move into the timelessness of presence, awareness, and stillness, love will be the outcome and can include profound sexual healing of past wounds. In order to experience this, basically the man goes in consciously and using lubrication, gradually traversing millimeter by millimeter as deeply as possible into the upper reaches of the vagina. He stays there not in tension but in relaxation, and sustains the penetration without moving. Eye contact (receptive vision) in these moments is very important. Timelessness arises and allows the bodies to go through a deepening of energetic exchange. Through sustained penetration in awareness, presence, and relaxation, a woman's receptivity is amplified, and there is a balancing of the entire energy system.

BODIES HOLD CELLULAR MEMORIES

It's no secret that modern mind/body science is now confirming that the body holds memory. An organ taken from one human being and placed into the body of another has an impact on the thoughts and bodily urges of the recipient, implying that an organ itself has cell memory. By the time a woman is menopausal, it is possible that she has endured some level of emotional, physical, and psychological pain on account of her life's sexual experiences. All of these leave an imprint in the cells of the vagina, surrounding tissues, and pelvic area.

There can be both physical and emotional scarring anywhere in the vaginal canal. For the menopausal woman, there can even be scarring from intercourse simply because the vaginal walls are thinner, which can create immense pain for some. More on that in the next chapter.

The cervix itself may have scarring from any number of issues, such as the removal of cervical tissue, biopsies, freezing of tissue for treatment of cervical warts, or scraping and suctioning of the uterus after miscarriage or abortion. A woman may also have experienced cervical tears from childbirth—from manual dilation, pushing prematurely, or having exceptionally large babies. Endometriosis and inflammatory diseases, as well as sexually transmitted or untreated bacterial or viral infections can leave scarring. Pap smears done without sensitivity for women whose vaginal walls have thinned can cause scarring along the sides of the canal.

There seems to be no end to what can happen in this small, sensitive region of a woman's body. Of course not all women who go through these things have scarring or feel any pain at all. And as with other parts of the body, the vagina has an unending capacity to heal. Simple, gentle finger pressure and holding still on these places can help to break up the scar tissue, but we suggest that if you have a partner, the best tool for this task is the penis itself. The end of the penis is soft, silky, and sensitive, and when a man directs the healing life force through his penis to any part of a woman's vagina, profound healing results. This truly can be considered a noble task. It is clear, therefore, that making love in relaxation holds great potential in clearing pain and memories held on the cellular level.

Pain as a Doorway to Healing

Making love slowly and consciously may bring up pains from the past for either partner. If you are aware of emotional wounds and physical scarring, you may decide you'd like to devote a few hours of your love-making to healing. When you begin to make love slowly, it may also draw forth some of these tensions and pains. This is not something to be distressed about but to welcome. It means that the cells are releasing old tensions and suppressed emotional memories. You may not even know what they are, but tears start to flow. You don't need to search with your mind for what it is or what it means; just let it be. There is such sweetness, such a closeness that occurs between two people when this level of intimate healing happens.

As the receiver, if you feel pain anywhere along the vaginal canal, including at the entrance, try not to jerk or pull away, just gently say to your partner, Can you please pull back the penis just a "hair's

breadth"—one to two millimeters? This fraction of space is very important because it takes the pressure off the pain and allows for the release
of tension. Both of you stay there with your presence. It's helpful if the
man, if he wishes to participate in this way, visualizes sending healing
light and love from his penis to the pain. For women, imagine softening
and relaxing the cells in that area. Take a breath. Soon you will feel the
tissue giving way and the tensions being dispersed.

You may then find another area is calling, so direct your lover to
that place and follow the same steps. Eventually, when the "work" is
done, the penis will take a rest and may even go soft. At this point,
allow whatever the bodies want to do without intervention. After lovemaking like this and if you practice deep, slow, sustained penetration
regularly you will be amazed at the transformation within you. Love
amplifies through this process. Men become more masculine and loving, and women more feminine and loving. This is without any goal or
seeking. It's a by-product of simple awareness and presence.

⏏ Self-Healing Massage

You can self-massage by using sensitive pressure on any part you feel
needs it, and from time to time, release the pressure with two or three
breaths and then return with gentle pressure using your finger tip. Evening
primrose oil may soften the cervix as it contains prostaglandins, which
are hormone-like substances that assist in the healing of tissue damage
or infection. Some practitioners are trained to release scar tissue by
massaging internally. Make sure you choose a practitioner carefully, and
find one who has integrity and is well trained, such as an Arvigo practitioner,
as mentioned in chapter 11 where more information is given. We discuss
sexual healing in more depth in chapter 9.

LISTEN TO THE CALL

Women in our retreats report a profound shift in their whole idea of
sex, and indeed their whole sense of themselves is transformed through

being interested in sensitivity rather than sensation. The call here is simple and relaxing. It is for you to deeply trust your feminine body. Be willing to shed the constraints and restraints put upon us as women to be something or someone in sex. When you just show up deeply in tune with your own instinctiveness, you simply are wild and natural. And remember, wild does not mean doing something special or producing some particular kind of behavior. This quality of "wildness" rises through being at home in your body just as it is! You continuously, reverently, and consistently drop back inside your very being, using the body as your bridge to your inner world, the source of your senses and sensuality. It is the bridge to your aliveness, the bridge to your heart, and the bridge to what perhaps you have been seeking all along. When you find that place inside and move from there, everything changes. You start to love yourself in a way that you may have never before felt. Life starts to change. A newborn sensuality emerges from deep within your bones without effort of doing.

Instinctive Movement

Choose music that is evocative and slow. In a grounded standing position, close your eyes, take a breath, and sink back into your body. Feeling your feet anchored on the floor, allow your body to relax and soften. Have the intention to allow instinctive movement to arise within your body, and then wait for any impulses that move your body. It could be a hand that starts to move, you may sway slightly, or your body may begin curling and unfurling. Whatever comes, let it be a meditation from stillness into movement. Do this for the duration of the music piece and then be still, standing, sitting, or lying down. Observe how you feel. Observe your inner experience. Relax and notice the aftereffects of this exercise.

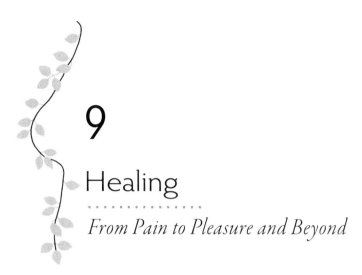

9

Healing

. . . .

From Pain to Pleasure and Beyond

THE PREVIOUS CHAPTER DEALT WITH the healing and purifying effects of sex when the power of awareness is incorporated. This chapter addresses more specific issues.

A woman may first notice her body changing during the perimenopausal stage, the ten or so years leading up to menopause. One of the first silent symptoms can be painful sex and vaginal dryness. Pain during sex is medically referred to as "dyspareunia." There are so many medical terms for women's so-called disorders! For women of menopausal age, dyspareunia often has a lot to do with estrogen, or rather lack of estrogen being produced by the ovaries.

There is nothing more disempowering for a woman than feeling pain every time she has intercourse. It challenges the very essence of her womanhood. Pain and discomfort can cause a woman to cut off from her lower body and ignore it, just wishing it would all go away. This in itself can cause her to feel doubtful and unhappy. Pain is more proof that her body doesn't work anymore or is broken.

As we have mentioned a few times already, more than half, and up to 75 percent, of women experience vaginal pain and dryness during menopause. But women in their twenties can have similar complaints, which implies that the causes may be many and varied, and

125

menopause is not always the culprit. Causes can include hormonal imbalance, vaginal health (including candida yeast infections), thinning of the vaginal wall, lack of readiness, cellular memories, scarring as the result of medical procedures, misplaced uterus, and internal organs placing stress on the vaginal area, or not being able to open up on a body level or a heart level. Drugs such as antidepressants, blood pressure medication, and allergy and cold remedies exacerbate the problems. Really, there are so many possibilities it's a wonder we can have any pleasure at all! For someone who is always dealing with pain, finally being able to open to pleasure can be immensely healing for a woman's body and soul.

As we've mentioned, with conventional sex your body may not have had the time to be open enough or relaxed enough for the vagina to really be receptive, therefore the tissue is being stretched by the incoming penis before the vagina is ready. The fragile walls of the vagina can suffer tears that can be incredibly painful. To hear women say that every time they have sex it feels like they have a knife cutting into them, and that some even bleed, is horrifying. One could ask oneself, Why put yourself through that? And this suffering just shows how programmed we are to want to please, as there is no pleasure in this in any way. Indeed, a man worth his weight, so to speak, would never want you to be in pain, especially through his being inside you. No matter her age, when pain is anticipated a woman's body will contract and become tense, even with the very thought of sex or making love. This tightening happens unconsciously. Even if she wants to be open, the body contracts to protect from pain. It is natural. The body has its own intelligence.

For a woman in this situation there is also a deeply buried subconscious fear of man and his power in sex and possible overbearingness. Often a woman feels she cannot match it or receive it, and feels overwhelmed. She fears an erect penis inside her because it means pain. As much as a woman and her whole body may want intimacy with her partner, the pleasure is mixed with anticipated pain. This is very disturbing for the psyche and body, and will invariably cause her to feel insecure and possibly unworthy about sex. She may compare herself with other women for whom this is not an issue. It can happen at this point that a man gets fed up and leaves for another woman who can satisfy his desires more easily. Or he closes down to keep things harmonious. Or they go about their lives in a kind of "closed door" way, where they live in the same house but no doors are open, literally or otherwise.

Sadly this is the scenario for numerous couples who do not have the information to understand their bodies at the deeper energetic level.

THINNING OF THE VAGINAL WALL

With the estrogen levels dropping during perimenopause, the vaginal walls can thin, causing less lubrication, risk of vaginal tears, and increased risk of vaginal infections. There may also be an increased level of urinary tract infections and/or urinary incontinence, as the urinary tract including the urethra also needs estrogen for tissue health.

Moisturize with Hormonal Creams

Some women who do not want to use traditional hormone replacement therapy (taken orally) find that a bioidentical estrogen (estriol) cream applied locally can work wonders for both the vagina and urethra. The cream can help your vagina feel moister, plump the tissue walls, and make them more elastic. Be careful if your breasts start to feel full, or your nipples hurt. This means you are taking too much and should reduce the amount you are using. Consult with your medical practitioner. Hormone replacement, bioidentical or otherwise, is powerful and it's important to use it with respect.

There are many alternatives for women these days to help reduce vaginal dryness and pain, which are easily researched via the internet. Women and men have been having sex for thousands of years, yet it is only in the last fifty years or so that hormone therapy has been introduced. As covered in chapter 2, many women have been greatly relieved of various symptoms through bioidentical hormones, which are molecularly identical to the hormones created by the human body. Some bioidentical hormones have been FDA approved, but not all.

Testosterone hormone therapy by itself is being touted as a way to lift a woman's libido. But this may be a superficial response, and perhaps not so holistic, as it doesn't take into account how a woman's body naturally opens in the ways we have discussed. Nor does it take into account the significance of progesterone, which is called the "mother of all hormones," because it acts as a precursor to all other hormones essential for women's health (including testosterone and estrogen), as explained in chapter 2.

Many findings indicate that adequate levels of balanced progesterone and estrogen can solve significant discomfort, without having to take testosterone. In our research we found both Leslie Kenton's book *Passage to Power: Natural Menopause Revolution* and Dr. Christiane Northrup's *The Wisdom of Menopause** to be comprehensive resources that explain menopause and the functioning of hormones in easy-to-understand language, and offer sound advice on hormone therapy, nutrition, and nutritional supplementation.

Hormonal balancing is a very delicate process. We are part of nature and nature does have remedies for all ailments or imbalances. You may wish to use some of the excellent herbal remedies available either over the counter or from your trusted practitioner, but the direction a woman wishes to take in her hormonal supplementation or remedy is a very personal choice for each woman, as mentioned in chapter 2. We recommend having hormones checked and speaking with a health care provider or doctor about the alternatives.

---

*Leslie Kenton, *Passage to Power: Natural Menopause Revolution* (London: Random House, 1995); and Christiane Northrup, M.D., *The Wisdom of Menopause: Creating Physical and Emotional Health during the Change* (New York: Bantam Books, 2012).

PRACTICAL TIPS FOR HEALING
VAGINAL PAIN

Lubricate with Organic Oil

Raw organic coconut oil is magic and when used frequently seems to plump up the tissue in the vagina over a very short period of time. You can freeze little strips of it and use about a thumbnail sized piece like a pessary (a small soluble block) that is inserted before or during making love. The body melts it perfectly and it seems to protect the walls of the vagina. There is almost no pain, providing one is aware enough to have a conscious entry of the penis. Coconut oil also has antibacterial and antifungal qualities, and seems to balance out the environment of the vagina for some. Apply a small amount first to check that you are not allergic. Walnut oil is also very good, as is pomegranate oil or even pomegranate pessaries if you can find them. Each woman must find what works best for her . . . what suits one may not suit another.

Stress and Tension

Stress plays a huge part in the lifestyle of all Westerners and affects not only the regularity and rhythm of making love but also the very bodies of the lovers. Stress and tension can manifest in all parts of the body, including the vagina. So it helps to make the time to wind down and consciously relax your bodies, and in particular the vagina, before making love. It might sound strange but you can use your awareness to actually direct any part of the body to relax, and the vagina is no exception.

Take Time before Entry

As mentioned, one big reason for pain is that a woman's body is not ready. Be unhurried in your approach, giving plenty of time for the transition to making love. Resting the penis at the entrance of the vagina is a very relaxing and peaceful way to begin and allows you and your vagina to soften and relax. Wait for the readiness of your body. Women need to guide the timing and slowness (millimeter by millimeter) of entry. Remember, it helps for men to allow the first erection of the penis to go down and then wait for it to return, as it will have a different quality, will be less excited and tense, and will introduce the possibility of being more present.

Prepare Yourself for Lovemaking

The most powerful and simple way to prepare yourself initially is to remember the significance of the energy-raising pole of the breasts. Hold the awareness, melting into them from the inside as in the breast meditation in chapter 7. The general idea is not to stimulate the nipples but more to connect with the actual internal tissues of the breasts. Try not to be goal oriented or tense about it, because that will have an impact on your body. Trust the intelligence of your body. Once you bring your openhearted loving presence to your breasts, the pleasure will spread in its own time, opening and preparing the vagina to receive.

You may or may not feel like making love. There is no right or wrong, just different bodies, with different histories, different makeups, different hormones, differing health, and differing ages. You are unique in your expression of the feminine; we are all different, yet so similar as well. So if you are not feeling like making love, accept it. Don't disappear down the rabbit hole of despair thinking you are less than, deficient, or failing as a woman. Now that you know your body is simply not yet awakened, you can relax knowing all you have to do is create the environment for it to come to life. Like the seed, you are power-packed with the potential of pleasure, of awakening, of love, of having a meaningful energetic exchange that can transform you and your experience with another. When you begin to understand the healing power of sex and how the female system truly opens, you will find it is worth being adventurous and experimenting, even if you don't feel lustful. In fact, not feeling lustful or "horny" can be to your advantage. Sometimes the resistance to making love is actually the resistance to being in the present, so on that level it's good to challenge your patterns of resistance. The bodies are always happy to make love, but the mind sometimes raises objections.

Gently Heat the Genitals

For millennia, women through the ages have prepared their bodies and vaginas for lovemaking. It may seem that we are focusing on the vagina here instead of the breasts, through which a woman's body opens at a deeper level, however there's no harm in giving the vagina and the surrounding tissue a little assistance and support. Arousal readiness requires the blood to circulate in that area, so gently heating the tissue is wonderfully nourishing. It feels soothing and relaxing. You can lie down with a very moderately heated wheat pillow pack placed between your legs. Comfortably rest it there, feeling the beautiful, soothing heat penetrate your vulva area. While the warmth is gently penetrating, you can cup your hands under your breasts or tune in to them from the inside.

Bathing Brings Warmth

Taking a bath before making love is a beautiful transition from a busy day. It allows you to rest and regenerate while gently warming the whole pelvic region. You may want to add some essential oils, such as lavender and sage, to your bath. Epsom salts (or magnesium chloride crystals) can be added, to help draw toxins out of the system and aid relaxation or release muscular tension. All bodies could do with more magnesium than we give them. If you have the right kind of tub, or even a bath filled to a shallow level, sitz baths are wonderful. A sitz bath means you rest your pelvis in warm water, bathing and soothing the lower realms. It is very nourishing and cleansing, and restorative for all the pelvic organs.

A retreat participant who shares her story below had struggled with vaginal discomfort and the condition of lichen sclerosus, which causes chronic itching of the vulva or anal area. The skin can become pale, thickened, or crinkled, which is why it's called "lichen."

ONE WOMAN'S JOURNEY

I'm writing to give you updates about my lichen sclerosus and inflammation, burning, and discomfort in the vagina. I am very pleased with myself as I continue with healing. Recently I am able, with soft and slow entry and without any coconut oil as a lubricant, to enjoy my lovemaking. I am feeling more "lush," I suppose. However, usually I do use coconut oil and it's a wonderful help for me, as entry is more comfortable. It's a continued healing. . . . I am working on my personal history for my healing. I can, however, always thank you for tutoring in the slow and cool lovemaking style as it is the only possible way for me to be able to make love with my husband. How sublime! We usually make love once a week—like homework—and the support for our relationship is fantastic. So life is grand and wonderful. I am so grateful and in awe at what my body can heal.

A Healthy Diet Can Lessen Symptoms

It is no news that nutrition will improve the functioning of all of the body's functions, including hormone production. A diet rich in vegetables and whole foods will often lessen symptoms. Some women have found that a complete break from sugar, even for a few days, has eliminated pain in the vaginal tissue altogether, as well as hot flashes. You may also find that an Ayurvedic diet designed to balance your body type can be beneficial, avoiding heat-inducing foods such as chilies, cayenne, and black mustard. Consulting a nutritional doctor or natural therapist who has a proven track record with menopause and female issues is strongly advised.

RISING TO CREATIVE SEXUAL POTENTIAL

Once woman experiences sex without pain on an ongoing basis, when the environment in her vagina has balanced and relaxed, she recognizes that she can meet man more easily. She is in a position to freely receive man, knowing the advantage of having a wide, receptive vagina and that there is no need to tighten, as happens in conventional sex. Her receptivity is not passivity; it is a "drawing," magnetizing force.

A relaxed vaginal environment becomes like a soft, velvety cushion, an invitation for man's energy, which significantly increases sensitivity for both partners, leaving them free to fully experience the potential of this exchange. With this awareness a woman naturally embodies her authentic receptive power. When a woman finally experiences and thus knows unequivocally in her heart and in her body that she can trust and fully receive and absorb male energy without pain, it is extremely uplifting and healing. A deep tension and anxiety in her relaxes and transforms into vitality. She glows. She rises elegantly to her creative potential. The life force now can move through her. She feels strong, radiant, capable, confident, and is gracefully feminine.

Whether or not a woman has a partner, she can meet life and masculine energy from a very different place, a more receptively empowered feminine place. This exponentially increases her self-esteem and brings a newborn confidence in her body and in her capacity to love. This radiates into her outer life in the form of inspiration, work, and relationships. Women often report having great bursts of creativity or more easily flowing into long-awaited tasks after slow lovemaking, proof that the sexual force, when moved upward through the body, actually is life-giving. This is greatly healing and deeply relaxing for a woman. For someone who has endured a lot of pain, finally opening to pleasure can be a welcome relief, one that often brings healing tears of joy.

A Little Yoga Every Day

Yoga helps calm the endocrine system, strengthens bones, relieves fatigue, and promotes general well-being. Remember that bringing some simple postures into your daily life has a cumulative effect on your system.

There are many yoga poses that help support the body through menopause by increasing circulation in the pelvic area. Because a woman's journey through menopause will be governed largely by lifestyle and imbalances, yoga can be a beautiful way to relax, recharge, and nourish the body.

So take fifteen minutes out of your day to bring these lovely yoga poses into your daily routine. They're great any time of the day to balance your whole system, and particularly relaxing before lovemaking or at bedtime.

Supported Bridge Pose
(*Setu Bandha Sarvangasana*)

This pose offers support for the ligaments of the uterus, as it helps to reinforce the muscles around the perineum and anal muscles. It is very good for the bladder and uterus, and for bringing blood supply to the generative organs. It helps to balance the thyroid glands, can be cooling for hot flashes, and helps relieve erratic mood swings, tension headaches, and depression. It's also helpful for regulating blood pressure, relieving anxiety, and encouraging sleep.

Set up props so that your legs are resting as shown. If you relax your legs out they will fall to the side. So this pose requires the legs to be slightly active, yet not so active that you are tensing. Find the balance.

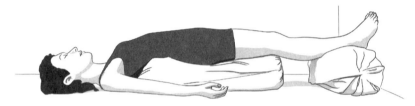

Fig. 9.1. Supported Bridge Pose

Supported Butterfly Pose
(*Supta Baddha Konasana*)

This incredibly relaxing pose helps to ease anxiety and stress as it tones and strengthens the adrenal glands and the pelvic floor. It may help to relieve symptoms of menstrual cramps and spasms or heaviness in the uterus.

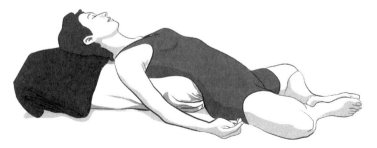

Fig. 9.2. Supported Butterfly Pose

Legs up the Wall Pose
(Viparita Karani)

This pose lifts and tones the pelvic floor, increases blood flow to your pelvic area, and calms the nervous system. Any inverted pose will help balance the nervous system and hormonal system, while improving circulation. This opens the chest and improves respiration, and is beneficial before sleep. *Do not do this pose while menstruating.*

To get into the pose, place a bolster a few centimeters from the wall and drape your pelvis over it.

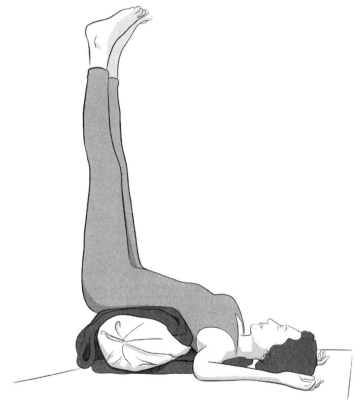

Fig. 9.3. Supported Inversion—Legs up the Wall Pose

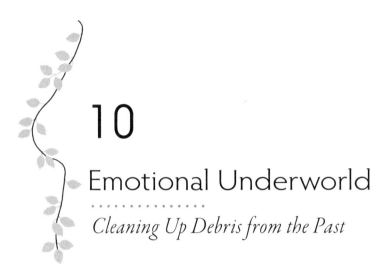

10

Emotional Underworld
· · · · · · · · · · · · · · · · ·
Cleaning Up Debris from the Past

BY THE TIME A WOMAN REACHES MENOPAUSE there has often been a watershed period when all that had been ignored, put away for another day, or not dealt with on an emotional level seems to have washed up on the shore. The bones of her past have been laid bare for her to sift through and decipher, and she can no longer deny some of the more difficult past occurrences to her body, her psyche, and her heart. In a way her past has begun to catch up with her. Her body has lived through girlhood, menstruation, perhaps pregnancy and mother-hood, and now she is on the threshold of another major transition. If she has been busy working or childrearing, what may manifest at this time is a level of exhaustion.

Women's bodies are regulated by cycles throughout this whole pro-cess. But the modern woman lives a linear life, continuing with her "doing" and taking little rest at bleeding time or prior to menstruation, which is essential for nourishment and replenishment. Women often have much that hangs in the balance as they juggle with satisfying the needs of all those around them. Because their natural tendency is to give, they may find themselves drained by responsibilities. Women's bodies are soft, vulnerable, and yielding, and at the same time resilient and powerful enough to go through childbirth. In generations long gone, and in traditional indigenous societies, a tribe or village supported the elders and the young. It was not the sole burden of one woman to support her family.

This relative isolation has placed huge stress on the delicate hormonal balance of the modern woman. If a woman's parents are still alive, they are aging too and she may have to step up to care for their growing needs. If she had children in her late twenties or early thirties they will be in the demanding teenage years and need a lot of guidance and attention. Therefore by the time some women are in their fifties or sixties, they may feel "sandwiched" by the demands of looking after elders while caring for the young. It can be a demanding and intense period, especially if there is prolonged illness or disability. For the woman who has chosen to have children later in her life, there are the high demands of parenting smaller children while going through the transition of menopause. And women who have been unable to have children, or chosen not to for various reasons, may be dealing with grief or sadness. Life stressors take their toll and cannot be avoided.

All of the above can easily intensify a woman's emotional world, creating a cloud that hangs as a layer of tension over her whole body and infiltrates her being, affecting her mental capacity to handle even the simplest of things. Layer on top of that the brain's scrambling to draw estrogen from the adrenal glands and elsewhere, as explained in chapter 2, causing increased anxiety, hot flashes, and so on, and there's a lot happening.

THE GIFT OF FEELINGS AND EMOTIONS

If there has been no opportunity in the past to really deal with some of the more challenging times, buried memories can emerge during this menopausal stage. If you are willing to allow any arising feelings, this can be a precious gift that invites you deeper into your heart and your being, and that will nurture your growth and maturity. When things start to filter to the surface, it is a time to clean up the debris of the past and find the hidden treasures within. It is time to reveal and heal. Addressing the past is imperative because when ignored, these tensions have an impact on your emotional world and can have disastrous effects on relationships and the physical body. Some women may not be aware of this aspect, or it may not be relevant, however, many women we speak to have reported a surge of memories and associated feelings at this time.

At some point most women who have been or are going through menopause could probably pinpoint something, a time or incident that became so devastating, so heartbreaking, that they felt the need to lie low. It may have been a marriage or relationship breakup, a health wake-up call, the unexpected death of a loved one, a crisis within the family, or some other thing that made her stop and question, stop and reflect. When this occurs it can feel like a deep dive into the female under-world, the depths of the feminine psyche, and may demand attention as a matter of survival. Whatever the event or trigger is, it will ultimately give rise to a new understanding of a woman's self, her life, and her body. Only she has the opportunity to tend to her emotional under-world and clean up her past to make way for her own heart to heal, shine through, and continue forward with grace and power. When a woman closes her heart to past pain and wounding, not only do her loved ones never get to share in her radiant beauty and love, in the end it is she who suffers most. In closing herself down she denies herself the very thing that can help her heal.

It's natural after some very big hurts to guard and protect yourself against future pain. Although putting up a shield may stop unwanted future pain, it also limits your ability to receive love and open to this powerful center in your body. When a woman closes herself, love can't find its natural expression. She has shut down the one thing that will lead her back to aliveness: a happy heart.

When a woman's heart is armored or closed down, it can cause all manner of body manifestations, such as illness, accidents, misery, depression, loss of sexual interest, and general low self-esteem. Love in all its aspects—including forgiveness, compassion, and gratitude—has the potential to melt the wounds of the past.

MEET THE PAST WITH LOVE

Escalated emotions can wreak havoc on relationships and can be embedded in the past. For some, it may be necessary to revisit the past, to unravel, to sift through, to make sense of, so that the psyche can finally come to rest. For some this may not be necessary. For others, it is imperative for moving forward. You will know intuitively what is suitable for you. An important part of that process is to simply feel and "be with" the feelings, rather than wishing things were different.

In addition to her own life challenges, every woman has a legacy through her family lineage that is both positive and enriching, and negative and challenging. We carry our ancestors with us in our genes, in our very actions and reactions. We see this in our children. Even if a child never met her parent or grandparent, the woman she becomes may clearly exhibit habits and body movements that are identical to those of that unmet person.

When a woman can be aware of the unconscious aspect in her emotional reactions, she has the choice and the power to create change. Even if she has the most tender, loving man in her life, her past and the generations before her live on in her and are likely to show up at least once in a woman's relationships, if not over and over again. For example, she may find herself reacting to her partner in exactly the same ways her mother did to her father. Understanding her lineage can serve a woman's growth and expansion if emotions are dealt with in a constructive way.

If we zoom out from our planet and take a bird's-eye view, we can see that woman as a collective and a gender has been suppressed and largely dishonored throughout modern history. (In different ways, this is also true for men.) Our past has created a collective wellspring of accumulated sadness, disempowerment, deep rage, and feelings of injustice.

Add to this the feelings associated with conventional sex, unloving sex, and the violation of women's bodies through sexual abuse or harassment. Include the individual circumstances of a woman's own life (religious and/or cultural shame) and you have a hefty mix of sources for a variety of emotions and feelings. In fact, you can find plenty of reasons for a woman to be unhappy or discontent.

Yet now, more than ever before, women are rising: speaking up for ourselves and standing up for each other. As a collective we may not have been free but we are now emerging through an era where women are beginning to find their voice. As one woman rises to speak, it invites others to stand and share their stories. As we share our stories, we are united in the healing of them. But nothing changes if we remain victims of our past. Women have a responsibility to themselves and to their children—future generations of women and men—to change the course of history through healing their past and their own awareness of their individual emotionality in the present. Part of this change involves every woman taking responsibility for her own emotional world. It's natural to want to blame others, be they men or women, but in the end it is each of us who suffers through holding on. As women we have the opportunity to prevent unconscious patterns from being passed down the line so that those who come after us do not repeat the whole scenario again and again. Emotions are often the roadblock to a loving, harmonious relationship. We as women are encouraged to step above the automatic, unconscious reactions and take a different stand. How can we do this? The answer may be twofold: dealing with the emotions of our past and dealing with our feelings in the present.

EMOTION VS. FEELING

It may help to look at Barry Long's interpretation of these two words: "feeling" and "emotion." These words are often used interchangeably, as if they are one and the same; however they are two different worlds on an experiential level.

Feeling Arises in the Moment

Long proposed that a feeling is the initial impulse that arises, felt as a phenomenon in the body, often on a sensory level. Examples of this are heat rising, cold enveloping, a grabbing in the solar plexus, pain in the heart area, or a wrench in the gut. These are pure and arise and move through in the present moment. You can see an infant expressing pure delight, pure happiness, then pure frustration, pure fear, and then back to happiness a moment later.

Over time, depending on how children are parented, they may grow up being conditioned by their parents or caregivers to know that some feelings are not allowed, not valid, or not accepted in their family or culture. A child's basic needs are to feel safe, valued, and loved. If their caregivers threaten these three things, even without intention, then they will start to mold their behavior and repress their feelings to suit the responses of the parents. Anger may be an unacceptable feeling in a particular family, therefore the accepted norm is to neutralize and suppress any spectrum of this feeling, from frustration or annoyance to pure rage.

The child may even be punished for expressing the raw feeling. This incident becomes an imprint, indelibly marked as a memory upon the primal part of the child's developing brain. Similarly there may be so much suppression of feeling that even joy, overflowing and expressed in an unbridled way, may not be acceptable. So children learn to suppress feelings and condition their responses to secure the parents' love and care, on which they are utterly dependent. The suppression turns inward and creates secondary feelings of anger or sadness, grief or fear. All children grow into adult men and women attempting to have relationships with each other. However, the past lingers on in the emotional underworld of each one.

Emotion Is Unexpressed Feeling

Barry Long suggests that these suppressed feelings turn into stored emotions within the body and psyche. Emotions in this context are then unexpressed feelings relating to the past—feelings that came up but had to be swallowed and repressed. As you grow into adulthood, these tensions sit like little time bombs so that when your loving partner does (or says) something, even something small or relatively insignificant, it triggers the suppressed feeling that in childhood (or at any time later) was not allowed. Basically it is a memory with its roots in the past. But you are not aware of this level of reality because it lies buried deep within your psyche. You may not be aware that the fury you feel about the way your partner is talking to you may be triggering the memory of how your father treated you as a child, so you have an emotional reaction to him that is far greater than the incident in the present really warrants. And probably you don't understand why you are so reactive. When this happens you have become emotional, and it indicates that something from the past is playing into the present and causing a disturbance.

Essentially, emotions are stored memories held within the cells—cell memories that in fact can now be measured by science. Dr. Candace Pert, author of *Molecules of Emotion,** discovered that when feelings have been suppressed, it affects the cell receptors to the point where they close down and ultimately can cause ill health. She found that once an emotion was fully felt and expressed, the cell receptors opened again, leaving the cell to replicate in a healthy way. Therefore, it is extremely healthy and invigorating to be able to express or allow your feelings when they arise in the present, and to deal with emotion that relates to the past appropriately, as in the ways suggested below.

Recognizing Emotion

Can you remember a time when you were feeling great and then someone said something that caused you to completely switch how you were feeling? You went from feeling love to feeling anger, for example? Or

---

*Candace B. Pert, Ph.D., *Molecules of Emotion: The Science behind Mind-Body Medicine* (New York: Simon & Schuster, 1999).

you went from feeling connected to disconnected? Sometimes a woman will become so emotional when something triggers her past that she becomes irrational, almost as if she loses contact with reality. The reaction is often instantaneous and triggers the fight-or-flight response. It's helpful to know that in fact it's the primal brain, or amygdala, that is being triggered, and the phenomenon is not limited to women. This "original" part of the brain is the most primitive and is designed for survival. It was the first to be formed in primitive humans to help them survive in the world of predators. It enabled them to have fast reactions when hunting and to safeguard them when being hunted.

As a species, other parts of the human brain have developed for more sophisticated social and mental functions, such as the emotional center of the brain and the frontal cortex. Incidents that are threatening to small children, such as trauma, are stored in the primal part of the brain. So when your partner says or does something that is perceived as threatening, even if it is seemingly insignificant, the primal brain kicks in, letting your nervous system know to be on high alert. Then follows the sudden reaction of anger, lashing out/fight-or-flight/running away, or complete withdrawal, which can happen in a split second. Emotional reactions of this kind can shatter relationships very quickly. So if we want to nurture a relationship into the long term, we need to find a method to interrupt this reactive pattern.

The first thing is to notice the sudden change in your body and become a witness to your reactions. Stopping them mid-track is important, and this takes skill. It is important to be able to notice and recognize when you are "in reaction," and there are common reactions that most of us do experience upon becoming emotional. To make it easier to recognize emotion, following are some symptoms and indicators that can help.

Indicators of Emotion

We ask retreat participants, "How does an emotional experience *feel*? What do we experience in ourselves, our bodies, when we are in emotion?" The answers given in response to our questions are similar in each and every seminar. Below is a list that describes the experience when suddenly the level of emotion rises and feelings of love just as suddenly evaporate. Emotion is easily and immediately recognizable by the following attributes:

1. The sense of separation or disconnection from the other person, as if a wall comes down between you, or you feel paralyzed. You also feel disconnected from yourself.
2. It is difficult to meet the eyes of the other person, you avoid eye contact, or the other person appears to be far away in the distance.
3. You blame the other person for the situation or for your unhappiness.
4. You use the words "you *never*" do such and such, or "you *always*" do such and such; you talk about the other person, not yourself.
5. You become withdrawn and closed.
6. Your body feels contracted, paralyzed, numb, and sometimes has pain.
7. Your vision becomes narrow and cloudy.
8. You are exhausted, low in energy, and wish to sleep.
9. You are protective and defensive.
10. You experience abandonment and rejection.
11. You experience loneliness and a sense of being incomplete.
12. You are self-righteous and refuse to give up because you are convinced you are right.
13. You feel misunderstood or taken for granted.
14. You want to argue, discuss, fight, and challenge the other.
15. Your mind is very active, full of negative thoughts and doubts.
16. The themes occur in repeating patterns, same issue again and again.
17. You feel helpless and a victim of your situation.
18. Your outlook on life is hopeless and depressing.
19. You get tense and prickly (like a porcupine); the other person cannot do or say anything right.
20. The emotional state of separation/disconnection continues for a few days before a return to harmony.

21. You try to change the other person.
22. You want revenge by saying or doing unkind, unloving things to the other person; you are toxic.
23. You react from ego and pride.
24. You kick into an unconscious pattern and don't comprehend why you are reacting in that way.
25. The reaction will usually relate to some incident or experience in your past.

We can call the somewhat uncomfortable experiences listed above the "symptoms of emotion." Usually you will suffer many symptoms simultaneously, and you may even observe other symptoms to add to the list! From now on, when one or some of these symptoms are present in you, you will begin to have the insight that you are *in emotion*. That something from the past has come into play in the here and now, and has taken over the show. In a way it is as if you have been temporarily taken hostage by your emotions.

It is helpful to remind yourself repeatedly that when you are emotional, the situation has little to do with the present. The emotion is resurfacing in the present, of course, but you are disconnected from the present. There has been a dramatic shift in your perception as a by-product of the accumulated and unresolved past that every person carries to a lesser or greater degree.*

Emotionality usually has fear as the underlying experience, no matter what the symptoms may be. And as the ego, the "I," gets activated and assertive during emotion, the ego forms a screen over the heart, covering over any feelings of love that may have been present just moments prior. Any action that comes out of this disturbed emotional place will not have a positive effect on your relationships.

---

*Excerpted from Diana Richardson and Michael Richardson, *Tantric Love: Feeling versus Emotion—Golden Rules to Make Love Easy* (Arlesford, Hants, U.K.: "O" Books, 2010), 10–11.

Experience of Feelings

The experience of a feeling and the experience of emotion are really like day and night. Feelings, when they are allowed as they arise *in the present,* give rise to a completely different inner experience. We ask couples how they feel in themselves when they share from the heart, expressing their deeper feelings. Interestingly, the feedback we receive on the level of feelings contradicts the previous list of emotional indicators. The words given to describe the experience of express-ing a feeling are almost the opposite of the words given to describe the experience of emotion, and shows that the two experiences are definitely not the same.

The conversation goes something like this:

Q: When you truly express how you feel, when you share your deepest feelings, do you feel separated from your partner?
A: No, of course not, we feel wonderfully connected.
Q: Can you look your partner in the eye?
A: Yes! It's easy.
Q: Do you feel contracted and collapsed?
A: No, expanded and alive.
Q: Do you feel closed, protective, and defensive?
A: No, open, soft, and vulnerable.

And so on as we continue down the list of emotions, asking for the corresponding words to describe feelings when expressed/shared/allowed in the present. Responses from our participants appear below. Each emotion is listed as in the previous section, and now after each symptom of emotion appears the opposite feeling experience.

When you have allowed or expressed your deeper feelings the fol-lowing attributes come to the fore:

1. Instead of feeling separation and disconnection from the other per-son *you feel connected and closer. You also feel connected to yourself.*

2. Before it was difficult to meet eyes of the person; *now eye contact is easy.*

3. Instead of blaming the other person *you are acknowledging yourself and expressing/sharing your deeper feelings.*

4. You do not say "you never" or "you always" and talk about the other; *you say "I feel . . . " and talk about yourself.*

5. You are not withdrawn and closed; *you are open and receptive.*

6. Instead of the body becoming collapsed, contracted, paralyzed, *the body opens and you feel relaxed, expanded, alive.*

7. Your narrow, negative, cloudy outlook *becomes wide clear vision and positive outlook.*

8. Instead of being exhausted *you are inwardly refreshed.*

9. Instead of being protective and defensive *you become vulnerable, open, innocent.*

10. You don't feel abandoned or rejected; *you feel self-accepting and safe.*

11. You do not feel lonely; *you feel complete, all-one (alone).*

12. You are not self-righteous; *you are understanding and self-revealing.*

13. You do not feel misunderstood; *you feel understood/accepted.*

14. Instead of wanting to argue and discuss *you want to exchange, share.*

15. Instead of being in the mind, thought oriented, and full of doubt *you are in your body, heart oriented, and full of trust.*

16. Instead of repeating patterns *things become spontaneous, changing.*

17. Instead of being a helpless victim *you feel empowered.*

18. Instead of feeling hopeless *you feel hope and trust.*

19. Instead of feeling tense *you can relax.*

20. It doesn't last for days; *you move on quickly.*

21. Rather than try to change the other person, *you feel acceptance for the other.*

22. Instead of getting revenge *you feel loving.*

23. Instead of reacting with ego and pride *you respond with heart and love.*

24. Instead of operating unconsciously *you operate consciously/with mindfulness.*

25. Instead of relating out of the past *you are responding in the present.*

Feelings Talk Only about Self, Not Other

Essential to the healthy expression of feelings is naturally talking only about the self, and not the other person. Sentences start with "I feel . . . " rather than, "I feel that *you* . . . ," which is a way of indirectly blaming the other person and is a sure sign of leaking your own emotions and not taking responsibility for them.

The usual resolution to the emotional stalemate reached in domestic arguments is that one partner will finally break down into expressing underlying feelings, vulnerability, insecurity, and pain. Invariably reconnection and togetherness is instantly created when one person gives up the fight, when the ego melts away from the heart and tears begin to flow.

The return to innocence, connecting to true feeling, has an alchemical effect on the situation, and the other person automatically lays down weapons and reopens their heart and arms. As soon as the ego, which temporarily obscures the heart, is put to the side, love will surface again. Love does not disappear in these moments of emotion, as couples so often experience, but gently waits shining behind the ego, radiant and ever present.*

HOW TO DEAL WITH BEING EMOTIONAL

We're not saying these steps given below are easy to put into action in the heat of the moment, but with regular use they will become more familiar and readily accessible.

1. Recognize and acknowledge that you are emotional.

The indicators above may help. It does take a little practice, courage, and humility to see where you are, but with practice, it definitely gets easier.

---

*Excerpted from Richardson and Richardson, *Tantric Love: Feeling versus Emotion*, 13–14.

2. Say aloud that you are emotional.

Have you ever felt so emotional that you have reacted in a way that you later regretted? We suggest that before reacting in your usual pattern, say out loud, "I am emotional" or "I am having a reaction," that you need some time for yourself *and that you will be back.* That is important! It can be very easy to want to hurt your partner, take revenge somehow, but if you want to shift your relationship in the direction of maturity and harmony, it's good to put into place some parameters for how you deal with high emotional states in the moment. Saying aloud "I am emotional" is often quite a challenge because we feel we are right and the other person is wrong.

3. Physically remove yourself from the situation.

If you stay with the other person arguing and discussing is likely to continue, and things can easily go from bad to worse, so it is wise to remove yourself from the situation and gain some distance. Try not to slam the door as you leave! Find a space or place that is private. At this point it can help to get in touch with your deeper feelings and gain some understanding of what the exact trigger was.

4. Move the body with intention.

If the emotions are overwhelming, we highly recommend that you move the body and *move with intention.* That means not to be half-hearted, to know what you are doing and why you are doing it. This is an easy way to allow unexpressed feelings from the past to be released. You may even notice the chemicals created by the emotion circulating through the connective tissue or fascia, the spiraling layers of fibrous tissue that stabilize and separate the muscles and other internal organs. Moving the body vigorously supports the release of these toxic traces, leaving you feeling cleansed and refreshed. Discharging in this way will serve to create some distance between you and the emotional reaction, as if "the story" has moved through and out of you. This allows for the survival or primal brain, the amygdala, to settle and for you to engage some of the more resourceful states from other parts of the brain.

Avoid rehashing the situation over and over in your mind, instead simply feel it as you walk, run, or move your body some other way, doing whatever you do with totality. Soon you are likely to notice that there is a change. It might transform to compassion, peace, or acceptance. Or it may clearly show you that a boundary has been crossed, but that you are now able to come back and speak to the person from a different stance, not blaming and reacting from the emotional child who is feeling threatened, but responding from the adult in a more loving, heartfelt way. You will also be more in touch with your own self and your own needs in the situation, which will help your relationship immeasurably.

5. Return to your partner.

When you feel you have completed the process, you are ready to return to your partner. It may take several hours. If you return to your partner and find that you have not reached a place of more refinement where you feel connected with yourself and able to connect with the other, that indicates that you need a little longer to navigate your way through the emotions. So communicate with your partner and say you need more time for yourself and will be back as soon as you can. The more you practice dealing with emotions in this simple way, the shorter the time span gets between becoming emotional and finding yourself returned to balance.

Communicating in a way that acknowledges both you and the other takes skill. If you'd like to explore this approach further, you may want to read *Nonviolent Communication* by Marshall Rosenberg.*

GOLDEN RULES TO MAKE LOVE EASY

Once again, these golden rules will probably need to be practiced for some time before they become your first response.

---

*Marshall Rosenberg, *Nonviolent Communication: A Language of Life,* 3rd ed. (Encinitas, Calif.: PuddleDancer Press, 2015).

1. Don't say to your partner, "You are emotional!"

There are a few definite no-no's when you take up this practice of separating emotion from feeling, and the first is that you *never* say to your partner, "You are emotional!" It's certainly a lot easier to see emotion in others, but transformation begins when you take responsibility and deal with your own emotions, doing your utmost to keep your territory clear.

2. Do not direct anger on another.

The second golden rule is about anger. This is an emotion that seems to erupt quite easily for women around menopause. Whenever you are angry it's important to *never* direct it toward a person. And you *never* direct it physically onto a person. You turn away and if the situation allows, scream and shout or yell and stamp your feet, or whatever. It is very healthy to allow anger to pass through you, and when anger is caught in its initial stages as a pure feeling, it will not last long; a few seconds and you're done. And you definitely will feel a whole lot better.

Additionally, fresh anger has a very different quality—it's pure and clean energy, whereas stored anger becomes dangerous because of its sour and toxic nature. So that's why it's important that you don't project anger onto someone; it's a strong vibration and too easily absorbed. Anger in its purity can save your life in certain circumstances; for example, a deep roar to repulse a stalker. The adrenalin rush gives you great power and force that can literally "blow away" your pursuer.

ALLOW YOUR FEELINGS

It becomes clear that the way forward is to let feelings flow through you *as they arise*. We tend to use the word "express" for feelings, however "press" and pressure are contained in that word, as if we have to do something, whereas it is simply an allowing, creating a passage, opening up to yourself. As a society and as children, we are not encouraged to allow feelings to flow, for fear of them being unacceptable. It is an art to allow your feelings, and one that will reward you and your relationships immensely.

The Art of Being True

When you give way to what is felt in the very moment you feel something, your experience is very different. As noted earlier in this chapter, the interesting aspect is that it will basically be directly opposite to experience when you become emotional. You will find that there is more spaciousness in your communication, more empathy for the other, and more deepened connection, first with yourself and then with your partner. It is clear that when you are true to your feelings your love will be able to flow, and any action arising from the willingness to be present to what is happening, in the here and now, will have a highly positive impact on you and your relationships.

Feel the Feeling Arise

Barry Long says that if we access a feeling in its purity, whether it be anger or sadness, it lasts just seven seconds. Many spiritual masters have confirmed this. Both of us have experienced this in the case of anger and sadness. However feelings of grief, for instance, especially if one has lost a loved one, are a longer process. Grief comes in waves, sometimes when we least expect it. But each time we give the grief space and allow whatever is there, it can lessen and we feel a lot better.

In contrast, Dr. Dan Siegal, author of *The Whole Brain Child*,* says that feelings last about ninety seconds. Seven seconds or ninety, it's still a short time! Then it does make us wonder how we can stay in anger, resentment, grief, or sadness, for example, for years on end. Simply, we are not taught emotional intelligence as children or as adults. If, however, we are willing to recognize/allow the feelings as they arise in the moment, even if some past issue is triggering them,

---

*Dan Siegal, *The Whole-Brain Child: 12 Revolutionary Strategies to Nurture Your Child's Developing Mind* (New York: Bantam, 2012).

then we will respond very differently; we will remain present, still, and fully feel the feeling.

Mind-body teacher Brandon Bays is the founder of the Journey Method, a guided introspective process that elegantly teaches you how to gently allow feelings as they arise, and allow memories stored in the cells of the body to be released. Thousands upon thousands of people around the world have benefited from learning the Journey Method and tools. She teaches that beneath the layers of feeling, *if fully felt,* are the true deeper feelings, and at the core of that, a deep peace can become available to you. To be still (as an alternative to moving the body) and just allow the feeling does take some skill and practice. See the recommended books section at the end of this book for more information on the Journey Method.

EMOTIONS AND FEELINGS
ARE NOT DISTINCT CATEGORIES

Although we have sought to define the difference between feelings and emotions above, it's good to remember that emotions and feelings are not two completely distinct and separate categories. Often when we are in an emotional state, after a while we might gain access to the true hidden feeling underneath, so in that way emotions can be a doorway to feelings, if you are responsible and aware. These may be the original feelings, perhaps giving you access to something you felt as a child but have never had the opportunity to allow to flow through you.

Witnessing and Observing

Initially with regard to emotions it's helpful to follow the five steps mentioned earlier. However, there does come a point where you can simply watch the emotional reactions. When we are fully present to what we are experiencing instead of following reactivity from the past and creating an escalating wave of emotion, this is very healing too. Witnessing means watching yourself, being the observer and bringing your awareness and intelligence to bear on the situation. So essentially you are fully allowing the sensations to flow through you, not running or hiding from them.

Emotions cannot be wrong because there are many reasons why we are emotional, especially growing up in societies where we are repressed and suppressed in different ways. However, *not* to recognize that you are emotional is "wrong" in the sense that sometimes emotional reactions can have lifelong and life-disturbing consequences, usually because of the toxic nature of the emotional state.

Low-Grade Emotions

Sometimes people report that they do not experience a clear distinction or shift between feelings (present) and emotions (past). It is more that they feel a little bit blue or generally disconnected and unhappy on an ongoing basis. This situation usually reflects a level of low-grade emotions, almost like a low-grade infection, lurking just beneath the surface. Symptoms of this low-grade state are quite clear, and it's very helpful to be aware of them because it is quite subtle and insidious and can contaminate your view of life. If you find yourself complaining constantly, this is a symptom of low-grade emotion. If you find yourself generally spiky or prickly or bristly or thorny or sharp in reaction or relation to other people, this is a sign that there is an overload of unexpressed feelings in the system. Or if you find that you are a bit testy in your exchanges, and deliver charged or pointed comments that carry a low level of toxicity intended to hurt or disturb or "get at" the other person, this is a low-grade-emotion symptom. Or you may say one thing but your tone of voice is intentionally conveying and delivering a completely different message. Another low-grade symptom is when you notice your mind is continually filled with blaming and negative thoughts, usually about others, especially your partner. You may not be up front and directly blame him, but the mind is constantly mulling over the way he is at fault or not meeting your expectations.

The remedy for low-grade emotion is basically the same as the suggestion given earlier: move your body! And move it on a regular basis, doing some set of exercises each day, so that the buildup of general tension and negativity is allayed. As a society we have become relatively static and motionless compared to our forebears, who naturally moved a great deal in the daily tasks of chopping wood, carrying water, and so on.

SEX AND MIND AS SOURCE OF EMOTIONS

Be mindful of what you let in! Conventional sex can lead to women becoming very emotional. We may not associate our emotionality with sex, but if you consider the unhappiness, especially of women, around sexuality, it is a given that sex itself (or the lack of it) can cause a lot of emotional eruptions or swings. Not the least of these can be the by-product of a man entering into the woman with his possible pent-up anger, frustration, neediness, or lust, complicated by her not being ready to receive him. Because woman is the receptacle, his tension and emotions can be deposited into her body on a subtle energetic level, especially when there is male ejaculation. It is for this reason Barry Long's compelling advice to all women was *only* "to make love when there is love enough." This is *not* to say tensions are deposited every time a man ejaculates inside a woman, but it is something to be mindful of in relation to what they brought to the bedroom prior to making love. We may have wondered why sometimes we feel emotional after conventional sex, but when we think about it, *how* we are having sex could have a massive impact on women, men, and the collective. During our couples retreats we invariably notice that women's emotions, the ups and downs or hypersensitivity, quickly level out. Women become much more serene, content, and calm after just a few days of engaging in slow, loving sex. Men, too, become more centered, present, and loving.

Trust yourself when the door to your vagina will not open. It may mean there are some low-level emotions lying around that you need to address. There may need to be some communication between you and your partner, or you simply may not be sufficiently relaxed. Let your vagina have the time she needs and she will open perfectly. Remember, too, that bringing the breasts into your awareness will help to relax and open the vagina, and also give access to feelings held there. If not, then try again a bit later or the next day, but don't get emotional and give up!

CULTIVATE THE POSITIVE

If you want to grow in positive, nourishing, and uplifting ways it is very helpful to cultivate four fundamental qualities: cheerfulness, friendliness, gratitude, and compassion. Through our constant mind activity and thinking, we easily get a bit tense and negative (low-grade emotional) about so many things without really noticing it. Through remembrance or mindfulness we can begin to affect our psychological states and our bodies in a positive way. And this will impact the quality of each day. You just decide to be cheerful. It's as simple as that—you switch the light on. Walk around feeling grateful for your life, for nature, for your body, and pretty soon you will begin feeling uplifted. Begin to be a friendly person to everyone you meet along life's path, including strangers, and suddenly the world becomes a more friendly, embracing place.

⊙ Reflect on the Past in a Meditation

Reflect on a recent emotional situation in which you could have chosen to act more consciously. Play it back in your mind, pinpointing the exact moment you became emotional. Imagine what else you could have done. See yourself doing that in your mind's eye and then see another possible outcome, and how that may have occurred differently.

TRANSFORMING EMOTION INTO LOVE

Recently my husband went on a three-month hike through the mountains on his own. Along the way he slept with another woman, and he told me about this during our next phone call. I instantly became emotional and felt totally disconnected. I could not imagine it was possible to continue our relationship when he got home after the hike.

At this point I contacted Diana to talk about my situation and to hear what she had to say. The question she asked me—"Do you want to meet him in love or in emotion?"—set many things in motion for me. So while walking on my way to meet him three weeks later it was good for me to tune in to a meeting in love. And I am so happy to say it worked very well! We had a very beautiful meeting. In the moment when I first saw him I noticed that it felt in no way that he was inwardly "gone," actually he was totally there and present. We could share many things and find each other again. It also worked well that I did not need to push away my pain; instead I could feel it and let it be there.

It was altogether an interesting experience, to feel that I could be fully "in" love, and feel the pain at the same time, that I could tolerate it and accept it. This was new. Otherwise, I would usually get angry when my heart was hurting. I also tried to go toward my husband fully open and approach him with no expectations, thinking about everything he needed to do now to make things good between us again. I managed this also and I could let go of all my concepts and meet him very openly. This is also new for me because I used to hide behind my concepts so as not to feel my soft and insecure side.

Since then I have a very soft and open and loving feeling inside me, above all for my husband, and interestingly I feel much more "close" to myself and also capable of "shaping" myself better. But all this is very easy and happening without pressure. It seems to me that I am more creative with myself and with the people around me. Your suggestion has been really worthwhile for me.

I (Diana) am very encouraged by this woman's sharing, and grateful to her for her trust, and above all for her courage. And for having the capacity, and the awareness, to stand for the truth of her essence—love. The question I posed her during our conversation—"Do you want to meet him in love or in emotion?"—was entirely based on personal experience; it had been a question I had asked myself many, many times! I, like so many of us, have all too often felt "betrayed" by a man through his going with someone else. At a certain point, as I was becoming more conscious in sex and love, and aware of unconscious emotional reactions, I did my utmost to choose love in the actual moment of re-meeting the man in question. I consciously resisted going into the usual pattern of emotion and drama. Much to my surprise, I managed quite well and on each occasion, I was blown away by how love could arise in an instant! This encouraged me greatly, and the truth was that I was so tired of my old pattern. I had a real urge to throw off the chains that have burdened women down the ages—the restraints of jealousy and possessiveness. History shows that infidelity happens, and what more can we say? Or do? I can state with all certainty that the conscious and deliberate "choice" to stand for love, and not to sink into the seething quagmire of emotions, resulted in quantum leaps that established new roots in my being and supported me in untold ways.

During our week-long Making Love Retreats, both of us have noticed that when the information about distinguishing between emotions and feelings is given, a few days into the week, a palpable relaxation fills the atmosphere. Couples realize that they no longer have to doubt their love, or their capacity to love, or to maintain a harmonious relationship. They now understand that love is always present and in order to nourish and maintain love, there is a need to manage emotions and feelings in a responsible way. And in fact, after the retreats, we both frequently receive messages from couples, telling us that to have learned the distinction between emotions and feelings stands in equal value to the reorientation on love and sex that they were given. And the perspective on emotions has been central to maintaining a field of love and harmony. This "coming down to earth" and seeing love in its true perspective can go a long way toward creating a more healing and loving style of sex.

WOMEN'S SEXUAL SHAME

We are strangled by the rules and regulations of a society that is more interested in controlling sex than celebrating what God has given us through our bodies. The mind and its ideas about sex have become dominant, while the intelligence lying in the body is overrun, often to the extent that the body is thought of as something to be shunned, shamed, and somehow made wrong. Woman carries this shame of sex as a weight in her subconscious. As mentioned earlier in this chapter, along with her personal history, there is the collective history of sexual abuse, of misuse of a woman's body. This is certainly not to ignore abuse of men. However abuse of women throughout all cultures of the world is much more prevalent. The sad statistics in the modern world indicate that as a planet we are still living very much in the dark ages regarding sex. All of this causes both the psyche and the body to contract in relation to sex, the very act that gave rise to our life in the first place. For it is through the sexual act of woman and man coming together that we are conceived and born. That we may be born into feelings of shame only perpetuates the story of the loss of purity and innocence that we unconsciously bear within our very cells, even as tiny male and female babies. So it is possible when you start to make love more slowly that these deeply buried feelings of shame start to arise. Allowing them to flow through you is deeply healing and integrating.

The good news is that conscious, slow sex transforms and heals you. Emotions that may have been a huge thing in the past can dissolve in one single session of lovemaking. The potential for healing is boundless when a couple brings their bodies together in awareness and love. Old wounds can melt away, new feelings of ecstatic bliss and peace can be experienced. And the healing happens within the actual cells of the body. Therefore, the potential for both cellular healing and the healing of a woman's entire psyche is enormous if she is willing to allow herself to be vulnerable and participate.

Menopause is the time to collect the treasures of your past and let them be gently allowed to see the light of day. It may happen that a slower, more tender way of making love will bring to the surface all that has not been healed, all tension and pain, all that overlays your love. So if this happens, welcome and embrace all of it with your love and tenderness. Allowing some of these deeper emotions and feelings to rise to the surface will heal, balance, and harmonize your body, your hormones, and your relationship, and in particular your relationship with yourself.

One of our retreat participants shared how gentle lovemaking released a lifetime of pain for her:

We were trying soft entry and I just couldn't go there, so I just let the penis rest at the entrance of my vagina. Just that felt so vulnerable, but I also felt safe with my new partner. I had so much anger, so much grief at compromising myself so much in the past, trying to please beyond what was healthy for me. We lay there for an hour and a half and tears just fell and fell and fell. All the times of feeling shame and abandoning myself came tumbling through me. It was like they were just all leaving one by one. Afterward I felt so cleansed, so innocent, so pure. I'd never felt that before in my life about my body or sex. I felt whole again. It was so healing. And the amazing thing was that my vagina that I thought didn't work anymore was plump, moist, and overflowing. There was nothing wrong with me! I've really loved my vagina since that day.

WOMEN SEXUALIZED
IN A DOMINATING WAY

In our oversexualized, male-dominated society, being "submissive" is seen as weak and even dangerous for a woman. The conditioning to please, to keep the peace, to sacrifice herself for others, to abandon herself, to do the right thing, reaches boiling point at menopause. Some women have had enough of doing everything for others. They want finally to do so for themselves. They want to feel their own pleasure, to put themselves first for once—and understandably so. Instead of trying to please a man a woman may choose to become more manlike herself in her approach to sex, seemingly more powerful and more dominant. We ourselves observe this assertive feature increasing among some younger women and certainly in career women who have had to don a protective layer to exert their authority in a male-dominated business arena.

Some women's drive for sex is heightened through and after menopause. They are, in fact, hungry for sex and can use it as a way to dominate and gain or exert power over a man. Sometimes they have been so hurt in past relationships that they have vowed that they will take the power back to gain the upper hand.

Sadly, though, a woman's focus can be misplaced as she wields her power from a place of anger (due to past hurts and male conflicts) and domination, rather than from the spaciousness of love. Sometimes what emerges is the "hungry" woman. She is just "too much," too overbearing, too outward. She may be great to have around, very entertaining, but "not the type" for a relationship. She is overly demanding and focuses only on what she wants; there's almost a hungry attitude about her. Not only is she hungry in her personality, but also that hunger can be expressed in sex and manifested at the level of her genitals.

Emotional Vagina

One could say that a "hungry vagina" is an emotional vagina, one that is needy, that is not balanced and not in harmony with woman's deeper feminine qualities. And woman treats her vagina in the conditioned way and does a lot with it by squeezing and contracting it to make it "tighter" during sex and to create more stimulation and sensation. The vagina is an organ formed by extremely delicate tissues and is designed by nature as a receptor, however it is being stimulated through friction, over and over, and focused on achieving multiple orgasms, multilevel orgasms, and the multiple types of orgasms she has been told are possible. On a subtle magnetic level she is turning and distorting a receptive or "negative" organ into a false "positive," unreceptive organ and environment, caused through the pattern of going for high sensation and intensity, and at the same time rarely being satisfied or fulfilled.

When women fall into this category, they often change partners frequently as men become overwhelmed by them, cannot keep up to their standard or level, and feel somehow demasculinized. Men can sometimes develop erection problems due, in part, to women's misunderstanding that they must reach out and do or get something, a reflection of the conditioning received through conventional sex. A woman who is using sex in the self-satisfying domain is moving from one man to another seeking the sexual thrill of a teenager and not embracing the true, deep wisdom of the mature woman. Or she is torturing her man with accusations of his lack of "manhood." This unfortunate fellow is in a double bind. He knows he is not stepping up but energetically she has taken so much of the masculine role that he has nowhere to go. This woman may be outwardly powerful, but she is internally disempowered.

Distortion of Male and Female Qualities

It's important to realize that what we perceive in the way of "man" and "woman" are slight distortions of our essential qualities as a result of the many unconscious conditionings and pressures in our society. However, when we understand the qualities and forces that we are imbued with, then it makes sense that woman as receptive power, as the container, needs to fall into and establish her true place initially. As mentioned in the chapter on the Love Keys, receptivity in itself is a force and power. It does not mean passivity or submissiveness. In reality, the intrinsic dynamic flow of male energy can only come into being when there is a corresponding spaciousness of the receptive female force. See the tables showing true female and male qualities on pages 164 and 165.

Regaining Essential Qualities

The pathway back to her femininity and her authentic power as woman is through her willingness to put down the armor and invite or open up to her very own vulnerability and intrinsic receptivity. A woman may often have good reason to be defensive. Somewhere in her history there may have been a time or experience where she felt very disempowered. She may have been humiliated, shamed, rejected, or condemned, and in order to avoid feeling that again, she has decided to have the upper hand. Whatever the reason is, if she wants to change this pattern it will help her immensely to soften to herself, take the focus off her genitals, and develop inner consciousness through melting into her breasts.

This is what Barry Long calls "being passionately undemonstrative." She is utterly present, deeply passionate, yet also yielding to the innocence, purity, and simplicity of relaxation, from a place inside herself that is receiving, not wanting or needing. As she develops consciousness in her energy-raising pole, her breasts, the powerful force of her intrinsic feminine nature will unearth a natural attractiveness within her that is not forced. She may find a new softness and grace that is still strong yet not overbearing. Then female receptivity can be a powerful force! The curious thing is that once she is able to cultivate this awareness, she may find that as she enters into lovemaking, her man does not have the erection problems he once had. Now the energy emanating from his penis (and indeed his entire body) has a place and space to be received. Instead of two tense overcharged organs working "against" each other, the vagina is enlivened with receptivity. It becomes a complementary organ that has the capacity to absorb male energy; and through a woman's breast awareness and genital consciousness and resting in her own self, an erection can be elicited. In this way a woman can have a positive and powerful influence over a man's erection. A man can feel fully received by his woman in a way he may never have felt before. Through this awareness and embracing the natural forces in the body, great love can be shared or exchanged by a couple.

☞ Mindfulness and Self-Forgiveness Meditation

Reflect on occasions when you may have used sex for power or influence. Practice self-forgiveness for that part of you that may have fallen into this trap or made unwise choices in the past. Come back to your heart and breasts, and soften into your body, anchoring yourself in love. Inquire into what drove you to make that choice, perhaps a feeling of low self-worth or not wanting to be vulnerable. Be with the feelings that move through you with compassion; there's no need to understand their source.

TRUE FEMALE QUALITIES
VERSUS CONDITIONED DISTORTIONS

True Qualities	Conditioned Distortions
Unconditional love	Love with conditions
Pure energy	Hysterical
Electromagnetic field of attraction	Projects attractiveness
Appreciates inner beauty	Attached to outer appearance
Receptivity	Passivity
Loving	Jealous, manipulative, possessive
Softness	Weakness
Relaxed, nondoing	Inertia, laziness, collapse
Earth, manifesting creation, nurturing	Overbearing, interfering
Embracing	Overwhelming
Ability to surrender	Submissive, giving in, losing self
In contact with feelings	Emotional swings, sentimental, moody
Sensitive	Oversensitive, prickly, brittle
Nesting instinct	Obsessed with security
Intuitive, psychic	Suspicious, fearful
Enveloping	Sucking, taking
Sweetness	Hardness, stoniness
Silently strong	Masochistic, holding back energy
Connecting	Invasive
Trusting, allowing	Controlling, indecisive, lacking initiative
Connected to the universe	Spaced out, lacking personal boundaries

TRUE MALE QUALITIES
VERSUS CONDITIONED DISTORTIONS

True Qualities	Conditioned Distortions
Pure consciousness	Unconsciousness
Power	Abuse of power, domination
Presence	Absence
Strength	Hardness, violence
Clarity	Judgment
Assuredness	Aggression
Directed action, dynamic	Activity, restless, doing
Creativity	Achievement, ambition
Will	Stubbornness
Courage	Compensation, arrogance
Leadership	Control, politics, law and order
Protector	Patriarch
Authority	Authoritarian
Wildness	Brutality
Clear mind	Arrogance
Charisma	Sexual manipulation
Expression, articulation	Pomposity, uncouth behavior
Heartfelt, compassionate	Selfish, egoistic
Differentiation	Separation

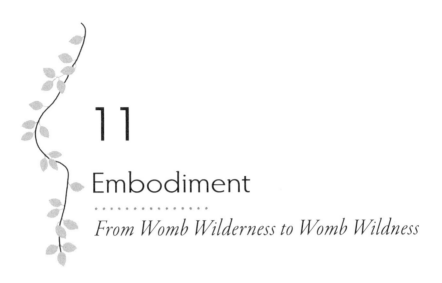

11

Embodiment

. . . .

From Womb Wilderness to Womb Wildness

FOR SO MANY OBVIOUS REASONS there is great sensitivity connected to the lower abdomen and, in particular for a woman, the womb. If feelings and emotions arise for you as you read through this chapter, take a deep, slow breath and relax your body. What we share here has been helpful for us. Your experience may be different. Remember that one woman's experience of menopause and womanhood is as different from another's as chalk from cheese. Just stay open, as this is a most delicate subject.

VALUING THE WOMB

Many women have little to no awareness of the womb, the uterus. The miraculous life-giving uterus with its capacity to hold space for the development of an embryo and growth of a baby is a muscular organ said to be, for its size, the strongest muscle in the body. It is so strong that it can contract and expel a full-term baby from a woman's body through the birthing process. A small, fascinating organ tucked up safely within the center of the lower pelvis between the bladder at the front and bowel to the back, it is shaped like an upside-down pear and is about the size of a fist in a nonpregnant woman.

Pound for pound, the uterus is the strongest muscle in the female

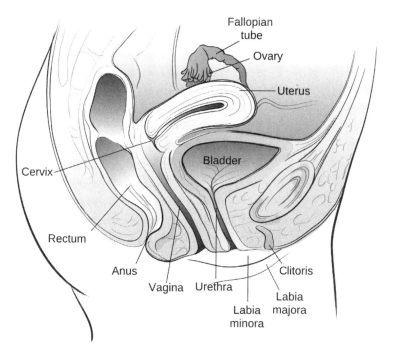

Fig. 11.1. Diagram showing placement of the uterus, ovary, bladder, and colon

body. The average weight of the uterus is from two to three ounces, and it's about three-inches long. It could be neatly held within the palm of your hand. When it fills with blood it can weigh up to twice as much, significantly swelling the abdomen just prior to and during menstruation. The uterus of a woman after menopause is smaller in size.

Because the uterus is tucked up safely in the lower pelvis, it is often unseen and not felt until we feel pain or become pregnant. Some women do not even recognize that a feeling of pain or fullness is in their uterus. For other women who have had no difficulties, it is simply rarely considered. For many, then, it is essentially a wilderness—a forgotten and untouched foreign region in the body and psyche, unexplored, neglected, abandoned, and sometimes even rejected.

Again, generally a woman's awareness is outside her body, not anchored within her being. Unless there has been childbirth or severe pain or a medical problem that can't be ignored, women go about their lives without really valuing this incredible organ and region of the body. It is also easy to understand that a woman can fall asleep to this area due to Western culture's lack of passing on important, essential, and helpful knowledge that is a source of inspiration for her and helps her relate to her body in a real way.

It is said that within the ovaries of an unborn girl are all the eggs she will ever carry, some 20 million, which is more than she'll ever need in one lifetime. This means that while innocently developing as a fetus in her mother's womb, she already holds the potential for her future children and her mother's future grandchildren; life begetting life, begetting life. Thus in the space of the forty weeks of gestation, there exist three generations at once: the mother, the unborn child, and the unfertilized eggs of the future generation.

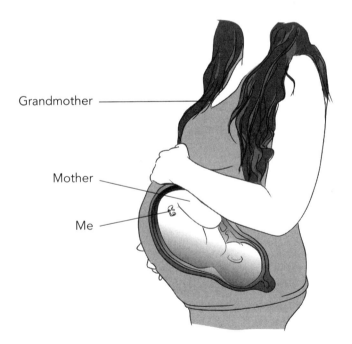

Fig. 11.2. Diagram showing matriarchal lineage: the thoughts, feelings and memories of grandmother may be passed down the line to mother and, in an energetic sense, to the potential egg from which you were conceived.

Negativity about menstruation, like menopause, is prevalent in most Western civilizations and can be passed on through generations, mother to daughter. Instead of viewing the monthly shedding of blood as the body's perfect way of eliminating excess buildup of the endometrium (mucous lining of the womb) that was ready to nurture a new life, it is seen as a defect, an encumbrance, an inconvenience to living. Modern-day advertising supports this inconvenience, telling women that they can essentially just put a tampon in and get on with their lives. Not often would a woman be encouraged to rest and take the time needed for this miraculous occurrence.

So from early on our culture has supported the ignorance of not only this precious organ, the crucible of life, but also of a woman's natural monthly cycle, the very process that begets life itself. Younger and younger women are suffering from uterine and ovarian-related issues—cysts, fibroids, and severe pelvic pain during menstruation or during or after making love. The medical history of the young woman becomes the history of the menopausal woman. In the same way, the attitude of the mother to menstruation, sex, and menopause has an impact on her daughters.

The uterus is a responsive, conscious, and spiritual organ suspended in place by seven different ligaments. Due to this ligament suspension, any imbalance in the ligaments can cause a change in the position of the uterus. Many refer to it as the center for a woman and it stores some of our deepest emotions and memories.

As women grow older many have been brought literally to their knees with excessive bleeding and uterine problems, and have had to choose removal of the uterus to come to some kind of peace, to be able to function in their lives, or as life-giving, life-saving surgery. This removal can be especially devastating if the woman is young and has not had children. Many women can feel it as a loss or failure of their womanhood.

UTERINE ENERGY CENTER

The reassuring news is that just as the biomagnetic breast energy is evident in women who have had breast-removal procedures, the same is true for women who have had the womb removed. The energetic of the organ is still very much there, despite its physical absence. However, women are more likely to avoid even wanting to think about this area as it can stir up shame, pain, suffering, hurt, anger, regret, despair, and even rage. Some have had not just one but multiple problems that might include cysts, fibroids, endometriosis, hysterectomy, caesarian births, stillbirths, miscarriages, traumatic birthing procedures, abortions, sexual abuse, or rape. If a woman has had multiple surgeries, she can feel it as an assault on her body. The scars feel like battle scars.

She never went out to war but she returns from this netherworld of medical procedures and unfortunate birthing stories like a war veteran. Alongside the emotional scarring and the memories are the feelings of failure as a woman, feeling like her body suffered abuse simply in the process of surgery. Such a plethora of mixed emotions steam in the melting pot of this potentially spacious organ, so adaptable and strong that it can distend and expand during pregnancy to accommodate a full-term baby. Deep in the subconscious of the female mind this mysterious organ is like an unexplored wilderness, to some an inhospitable place—a place that once visited through pain or trauma holds too much emotional residue and therefore is best left out of the awareness to get on with it all . . . to soldier on. This is supported by the mainstream medical world, that the womb is considered to be of no use once the childbearing years are finished.

Surgical removal of the uterus remains one of the most commonly performed operations in the United States. Both doctors and their patients have been taught that these organs are dangerous, at worst, or expendable at best. Though this stance is now changing rapidly, one in three women in this country has had a hysterectomy by the age of sixty. This is a staggeringly high number. Not surprisingly, hysterectomy rates are very high among doctors' wives and about 55 percent of women have their ovaries removed at the same time as their uterus to prevent the possible development of ovarian cancer, despite the fact that the vast majority of us will never get ovarian cancer but could definitely benefit from the hormones produced by our ovaries throughout our lives.

Your uterus, cervix, and ovaries all work together to provide your body with hormonal support throughout your entire life. They also share much of the same blood supply. When the uterus is removed, the function of the ovaries is affected even if the ovaries are left in.*

As with many areas of women's health, modern medicine with all its wonders has made women fall asleep to themselves, to their body awareness, and to their intuition about their bodies. Instead they allow an override of what they know in their bones to be wrong and place authority in the culture of a pill for this and a pill for that, a procedure for this and a procedure for that. At the same time these procedures can be lifesavers, and as wonderful as medicine is, it could rise to even greater heights if women were given their voice and full information about their own bodies. Only since the start of the health revolution have women been waking up to the fact that they can take their health into their own hands. It is no wonder, then, what with modern medicine and the conventional sex approach, that a woman is turned off to the idea of bringing her awareness to this area either physically or emotionally. However, this is where conscious, slow lovemaking comes to the fore.

WOMB WISDOM

Nestled inside a woman's body like a sacred secret, the womb can be said to hold a woman's deepest mystery. The womb is the body's birthing center. Hidden deep in the pelvic cavity it carries the very essence of creation, the potential of creating and gestating life, the ability to

---

*Christiane Northrup, M.D., *The Wisdom of Menopause: Creating Physical and Emotional Health during the Change* (New York: Bantam Books, 2012), 292.

harness and nourish life for the continuation of our species. The natural wildness of nature lives on through this amazing organ, whether she creates a new life or not. Yet this potent fact is bypassed simply through lack of knowledge and acknowledgment. With the worshipping of all things to do with the mind in our modern society, to even contemplate something buried within our bodies as something other than its biological purpose for woman to reproduce may seem farfetched. Christiane Northrup says, "The uterus is related energetically to a woman's innermost sense of self and her inner world. It is symbolic of her dreams and selves to which she would like to give birth."*

However it is through a woman's awareness and connection to her womb that she can find some inner ground and plant roots within her own being. There are more neural pathways in the womb than in any part of the brain, which makes it not only more sensitive but also more intelligent.

As we have stated previously, when a woman connects to her breasts as her dynamic and vibrant center, this awareness gives rise to a different quality. However when a woman makes the mistake of connecting only to the heart area, this can make her ungrounded and allow her to easily become overwhelmed by her emotions and fears.

For a woman to visualize grounding herself deep within her pelvis through her womb area (the *dantian* or *dan tien* or *tan t'ien*, as Taoists refer to it, loosely translated as "elixir field") gives her great strength and presence. From here she can begin to live freely from her own instincts, cultivating an inner power that can unleash boundless creative ideas, initiate and nurture projects, and grow her wisdom naturally, with no force needed. It's from here, along with the cultivation of a compassionate heart, that a woman can grow herself from girl reactions to woman-wise action. A feeling felt deeply and taken to the womb area can be transformed. The mind might fear doing

---

*Christiane Northrup, M.D., *Women's Bodies, Women's Wisdom: Creating Physical and Emotional Health and Healing* (New York: Bantam Books, 2010), 177.

such a thing, thinking it might hurt the body, but in fact the feeling/ emotion is transformed through this area and thus it becomes empowering and balancing.

Janet shares the following story about using her womb as a calming medicine:

I was feeling tremendous anger in relation to the lifestyle choice of a relative. I took myself away where I could be completely in private. Usually the feeling would escalate into many stories. Instead this day I chose to stop, to just feel the feeling. I imagined taking this rage to my womb. Instantly, I calmed. It stopped. It was like it evaporated. Quite soon after, I was able to return to the situation and continue dealing with it in a balanced way.

THE CREATIVE POTENTIAL OF THE WOMB

The menopausal woman, therefore, has much to look forward to as she embarks on what can potentially be one of the most fruitful periods of her life. If a womb has the potential to create human life, then it also has the potential to create, per se. No longer is the energy needed for creating babies, but this creativity extends to the rest of her life. Symbolically the ovaries can be seen as carrying the seeds of an idea or inspiration and the womb can be seen as the holding space for those ideas to take hold and germinate. Not all seeds/ideas need to come to fruition, and sometimes ideas come and go and do not grow into anything, just as the egg embeds in the endometrial lining of the womb and then leaves through menstruation. In menopause we can say that, metaphorically speaking, the energy is now being held within and can be reabsorbed and amplify the creative power.

As mentioned in chapter 2 on hormones, it is now being found that the ovaries and other parts of the body continue to create their own hormones, thus equally affording the woman beyond menstruation the potential for all the right chemicals she needs to move on into elder life.

It is how she lives in accordance with her own wishes that affect her most profoundly.

The womb itself is a receptive organ. As we know, when the egg is released from the ovaries every month it simply waits embedded in the cushiony walls of the womb, sending hormones out to attract the sperm. But it does not go and actively seek; it is the sperm that wriggles and thrusts forward to find an egg to penetrate. Thus the receptivity of the uterus along with the vagina gives rise to its inherent nature and informs a woman as to how she can consciously use her womb awareness in her outer and her inner life.

So this means that in lovemaking her attention within this area, including her awareness in her breasts, can give rise to an energy that amplifies something also untamed in her, a fragrance of woman as individual as she is. As she gently moves with the subtle rhythmic impulses of the womb and pelvis while making love, ecstatic waves of bliss naturally and spontaneously start to emanate through her. When a woman cultivates her sensitivity and awareness of her inner body, her "inner cosmos," she can palpably feel the effect breast awareness has on her womb.

At times she may literally feel it like a pulsing, the direct correlation of the "inner rod of magnetism" that was explained in chapter 3. So the womb can be felt at times moving and pulsing ever so subtly while resting in apparent stillness, in the same way that the vagina pulses. Natural and wild without restriction or tension, the receptive vagina and uterus are set free in the dynamic stillness of awareness. In lovemaking, if a woman consciously rests and relaxes in nondoing, she will notice that through its natural pulsing the vagina receives and draws the penis deeper and deeper within its chambers through its very own organic, peristaltic action—effortlessly yet potently taking his maleness into the warm, soft velvet environment of its cushioned comfort. So her breast awareness, while also bringing attention to the womb and vagina, will enhance her experience (as well as his) and help give her the confidence that in fact her body is a biomagnetic, bioenergetic organism and is working perfectly, menopausal or not.

In this way feminine sexuality at menopause is a vessel nourished by life and growing to fullness. Even a woman without a partner can know deeply within her being that this receptive potential is very powerful and in fact can be a great asset in receiving what she truly wishes to manifest.

ORGAN REMOVAL—THE DISPLACED UTERUS AND TENSION

The womb may, at times, undergo less-welcome changes. The medical term *hysterectomy* was derived in 1886 from the Greek word *hysterikos,* meaning "suffering in the womb," and the procedure was thought to cure a condition of extreme excitability unique to women (hysteria). This same condition was already regularly treated by physicians using manual massage of the genitals in the first century CE (presumably stimulating to release an orgasm); another remedy devised in the nineteenth century for the same malady was "vibration therapy." Unfortunately, however, hysterectomy won the day and has become one of the most frequent operations performed around menopause. Removal of the uterus can affect the pelvic nerves and blood supply, as well as the positioning of the organs around the uterus, and can affect bowel and bladder function. Any disturbance through surgery will create scar tissue, the body's natural way to heal and strengthen the area that was once very soft tissue, turning it into harder tissue to heal the site.

The whole pelvic area can be a storehouse of tension for a woman. The womb with the cervix at its entrance, at the end point of the vaginal canal, is not a body area that would seem to have/carry tension. Remember, we referred to this area as the garden of love in chapter 8. But the cells within any body part, tissue, organ, or muscle all carry memories. This has been evident to both of us in our own personal journeys, as memories have spontaneously arisen during conscious lovemaking. In the womb, cervix area, vagina, and entire pelvic floor region such memories can include birthing, miscarriage, abortion, medical procedures, or rape. Interestingly the ligaments attached to the pelvic

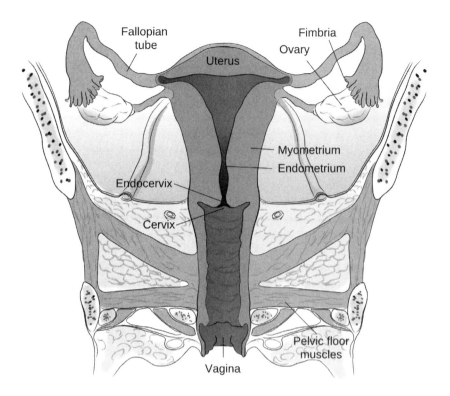

Fig. 11.3. Diagram showing a frontal view of the position of the pelvic organs and surrounding support structure

sidewalls that hold the uterus in place can also hold a key to some internal symptoms that arise. Males do not have these ligaments to hold their sex organs in place. Because the female body needs to be able to hold the great weight of a growing baby within its frame, powerful ligaments are attached to the pelvis, pubic bone, sacrum, and spine.

When these ligaments are contracted or overly extended, they can cause pelvic pain and, along with it, displacement of the uterus. If one side is tight and the other distended, this imbalance can cause the uterus to tilt one way or the other. When the uterus is in an incorrect position it can receive too little blood flow to the area and cause issues such as menstrual difficulties or pain, birthing difficulties, or unexplained pain in the sacrum or tailbone. It can cause further problems when subjected to high-impact exercise or carrying and lifting heavy objects during menstruation or pregnancy. Indeed, displacement can affect emotions stored in that part of the body. Also the elimination organs of the bladder and bowel can affect the health of the uterus. For example, an enlarged large intestine will invariably affect the placement of the uterus over time.

All of these, in fact any discomfort at all, will inhibit a woman's ability to feel pleasure in this precious part of her body. Any imbalance will inherently hold within it a lack of blood flow, a typical impediment to interest in sex and pleasure.

ARVIGO TECHNIQUE OF MAYA ABDOMINAL MASSAGE

The Arvigo Technique of Maya Abdominal Therapy is based on the traditional Mayan technique of abdominal massage. It is a very gentle, non-invasive, and effective massage that centers, lifts, and balances the uterus. It is named after Dr. Rosita Arvigo, who studied in a small village under "the last Mayan bush doctor," Don Elijio Panti, for thirteen years before he passed away at age 103 in 1996. Don Elijio treated women for all sorts of ailments in the abdominal region, from menstrual difficulties to fibroids, to prolapse and many more. He was internationally famous for his "folk chiropractic" traditional bodywork techniques, a part of a thousand-year-old oral tradition that continues to be passed down from one generation to the next throughout varied cultures of the world.

Done by professionally trained practitioners, Maya Abdominal Therapy involves a careful scooping-upward action from the base of the abdomen to the belly button. This helps to gently ease the tension in ligaments and allows the organs to come back into alignment. Dr. Arvigo is now based in Belize, where she teaches women how to perform the massage, and it is taught in the traditional manner—by word of mouth, woman to woman. In addition, there are now trainers in many parts of the world, including America, Europe, Australia,

Israel, and New Zealand, who teach practitioners how to perform the Maya Abdominal Self-Care massage.

WARNING: This massage must *not* be done if you are pregnant, have had abdominal surgery within the last six months, have cancer or pelvic inflammation, or wear an IUD for birth control. We strongly advise that you seek a trained Maya Abdominal practitioner in your region for treatment. The Arvigo website is in the resource section of this book.

Vaginal Steam Baths

The massage technique and vaginal steam baths (*bajos,* in Spanish, from "bottom"), also taught by the Arvigo Institute, form a very effective treatment for prolapse and organ displacement. Korean healers called *chai-yok* use vaginal steam for fertility issues to cleanse the uterus, not during pregnancy but to ready the uterus for pregnancy. It can help issues such as irregular menstrual cycles, ovarian cysts, urethral problems, fibroids (not to be used with heavy bleeding), endometriosis, repairing of scar tissue, organ prolapse, vaginal and yeast infections, and more. And in some traditions, vaginal steam is used to ready the vagina for lovemaking. It is a simple twenty to thirty minute process done with prayerful intention while seated over a bowl of warm water that has been simmered with herbs for five to ten minutes. The lower body is covered with towels so the steam does not escape. It is recommended to lie down for an hour afterward to allow the blood to circulate and to rest.

The Mayans used herbs from the forest chosen specially for that particular woman, as do Maya Abdominal Therapy practitioners. They use fresh organic herbs, *not oils.* Some of the common dried herbs used are marigold, lavender, and chamomile. An Arvigo practitioner prescribes what you need according to your symptoms.

WARNING: Steaming must *not* be used if you are pregnant, have extremely heavy menstrual cycles, are currently menstruating, or have a wound, sores, blisters, or any kind of active infection. You *must* do this with a trained practitioner. The steam should be gentle and at no time cause pain or burning.

Dr. Arvigo says the vaginal steam brings much-needed blood to the pelvic organs. The tissues of the vagina are porous and absorbent, and the warmth of the steam softens and opens them, allowing the medicinal properties of the herbs to infuse the tissue and bloodstream. You can find out more about the pelvic massage and vaginal steaming in *Journeys into Healing* from the Arvigo Institute.* Courses are being taught to pass on these powerful and effective healing practices, and some spas now offer it as a service. Here is a link to a clip of a Westernized "V Steam" at a holistic spa: http://bit.ly/2w6r8GE.

Pelvic Operations and Scarring

As we know, any kind of surgery that leaves scarring will affect the whole pelvic region as the scar tissue pulls on other tissue and drags it across places it normally would not be. This can create tension and strange referred pain/s deep in the pelvis. Scar tissue can be both inside and outside the body, as layers of muscle and nerve are spliced through to remove or lift a prolapsed organ into place. The Maya abdominal massage may include sensitive bodywork on scar tissue that may help to release some of this tension and soften the area. Maya abdominal massage therapists are trained to do intravaginal massage if needed as well as gentle healing touch for the pelvic floor, which can hold tension.

PROLAPSE—THE FOREIGN LAND

Unless a woman experiences the phenomenon of pelvic organ prolapse, the idea of an organ or part of the body protruding from the vagina,

---

*Arvigo Practitioners, *Journeys into Healing: Inspiring Experiences of Arvigo Practitioners and Their Clients* (Antrim, N.H.: The Arvigo Institute, 2014).

urethra, or rectum is totally foreign. A prolapse literally means to "fall out of place." As any woman who has experienced this can attest, it is a horrifying occurrence and takes a woman completely by surprise. This is another fairly common event that mostly remains unspoken among women, until one gets behind the veil of silence and embarrassment. A surprising number of women report prolapse, from ages as young as eighteen through to the seventies and eighties. If the womb is a wilderness for many women, the thought of prolapse of any abdominal organ could be a foreign land.

If a woman has not had much awareness in her pelvic organs, uterus, and so on, before she has a brush with prolapse, she certainly will need to let her body learn a new language—that of investigating both the causes and what she can do about healing it. This can most certainly affect her ability to open up to sex in the conventional style.

To explain more fully, pelvic organ prolapse occurs when one or more organs in the pelvis—the cervix, uterus, vagina, urethra, bladder, or rectum—shifts out of position, puts pressure on the uterus, and slips downward and bulges into or out of the vaginal canal. The symptoms are a feeling of fullness or pressure in the vagina or lower pelvic region, and a feeling as if something is falling out, somewhat the way a tampon might feel if it's not inserted properly. There may be a feeling of not being able to fully empty the bladder, leaking of urine, or complete incontinence. There may be frontal pain unrelated to menstruation, lower back pain, or difficulty in emptying the bowel. Symptoms can range from what seems like a urinary tract infection, slight bladder leakage, and discomfort to a full-blown incident of the organ dropping through the vagina or rectum. In addition, the lining of the urethra walls can fall through the urethra, due to the thinning of the tissue in menopause, which can be exacerbated by a lifestyle of straining or pushing in urination, being in a rush all the time, long-term stress, or heavy lifting. Similarly, the bowel can prolapse through the rectum and this can range from mild discomfort and difficulty emptying stools to a protruding inner rectal lining. Again, straining during emptying of the bowel may contribute to this problem.

There are multiple theories from many medical professionals about the causes of prolapse—various things that can happen during birthing procedures, birth itself, past health history, weak pelvic floor muscles, weakened internal muscles and ligaments in the abdominal area, or simply the aging process and lowered estrogen levels that cause the tissue to lose its strength and elasticity. It's good to understand that each woman's history is completely unique and her remedies for prolapse or pelvic discomfort can come in many forms. What we offer here is something that has helped women we know personally, and many women around the world. Any kind of persistent pelvic spasms or pain unassociated with menstruation should be investigated right away so you can be armed with the knowledge of what to do about it.

One woman was surprised to discover that she was suffering from a prolapse:

At first when I heard about prolapse from an older friend who had suffered for a long time with it, I am embarrassed to say I felt horrified to even talk about it and couldn't imagine how that could possibly happen to the human body, let alone mine. As fate would have it, several years post menopause I had a nasty coughing flu for six weeks. After that, I noticed minute urine leakage at night that was waking me from sleep. Six months later the day came when I finally became aware that I was suffering with it as well. Was it childbirth that caused it? Was it menopause? Was it the coughing alone? Was it weak pelvic floor muscles? Was it that I have always slouched when I sat on a couch since I was a teenager? I can't really say; perhaps a combination of all of these. It set me on a journey that led me to Christine Kent's Whole Woman work.

Christine Kent, founder of Whole Woman, Inc., is an American Registered Nurse who has dedicated much of her latter life to an in-depth investigation into the causes of prolapse, and her findings and remedies are creating a worldwide grassroots movement in its treatment. Her work is interesting and turns what we have known about pelvic organ self-care on its head. She says that there is no surgical cure for prolapse but the condition can be easily stabilized and occasionally reversed.

Kent believes that prolapse is a symptom, the result of a larger picture. She suggests the cause is not so much weak pelvic floor muscles but postural misalignment and the lack of integrity of the ligaments holding the organs in place, departing from the natural way the pelvis should sit. While the modern woman concentrates on tightening her stomach muscles and tucking her tailbone in to create the ever-desired flat female stomach of our time, she is compromising the very foundation of her body and its natural potential to live a future pain- or symptom-free life.

Equally, many teenage girls of today have stooped, concave shoulders, which sink the breasts and push the pelvis forward, bringing the whole structural alignment of the female into question. The thrusting forward of the pelvis causes a flattening of the lower back, a departure from the girl's natural spinal curve. This tension puts strain on all the internal ligaments, thus compromising the positioning of the organs, compressing them instead of allowing them to be held in their optimal position. Add to that the lifestyle of sitting for hours on end, as compared to our grandmothers or great grandmothers who would have been much more active in their average daily routines.

Christine Kent writes:

Human females in Western civilization are experiencing a dangerous evolutionary gap. That which at one time was unconscious and instinctive (that is, posture) now takes conscious control to maintain. In reality no one can do this work for us. We can travel from physical therapist to chiropractor to uro-gynecologist and back again, but in the final analysis only we ourselves can learn to live well moment to moment with the natural shape of our original design.*

---

*Christine Ann Kent, *Saving the Whole Woman: Natural Alternatives to Surgery for Pelvic Organ Prolapse and Urinary Incontinence* (Albuquerque, N.M.: Bridgeworks, Inc., 2008), 122.

Posture for Pelvic Health

Gone are the days of Flemish artist Peter Paul Rubens' women who lie lavishly across Grecian architecture and in hot baths, bellies hanging out and rolls of skin gracing the canvas. How luscious and beautiful these women were! Modern Western women have suffered a lot at the hands of the culture and customs of hundreds of years of tucking the tailbone under and pulling in stomach muscles. It's not so easy as one gets older, but some still try. Nevertheless there is a certain tension that is held in the solar plexus region, if this has been the default position.

⌇ Postural Self-Observation

As you read now, stand up and try it out. Suck in your stomach and you will notice that your tailbone naturally tucks under slightly. When you are mindful of this, you will notice how much tension it places on the pelvic floor, vaginal muscles, and buttocks. Even more than that, though, it places a permanent strain on the ligaments that hold the pelvic organs in place and can cause a lack of tone in other ligaments that are slack. Thus it creates tension in some ligaments and lack of tension in others, resulting in a lack of tone.

If we observe indigenous women's posture, such as African and Indian women, we notice they naturally stand upright with a slightly arched back, showing a beautiful curve in their spines. Their chests are high and their shoulders rest effortlessly over the pelvis, which enables them to walk smoothly and gracefully. The apparent ease of carrying heavy baskets and loads on the head are made possible by their very posture and alignment.

Children offer a wonderful lesson in good posture in the way that they naturally sit upright, as illustrated on the following page in a photo of Janet's granddaughter.

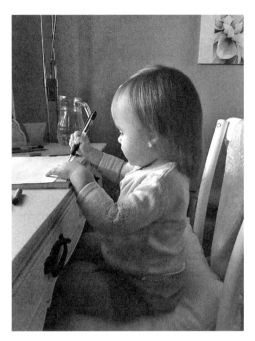

Fig. 11.4. Janet's granddaughter sitting at table
with natural upright back

Christine Kent,
Founder of Whole Woman, on Prolapse

Prolapse is not caused by childbirth, weak connective tissue, or weak pelvic floor muscles. Prolapse is a structural problem. It is the result of loss of the natural lumbar or lower back curvature, which is the natural female shape.

The loss of lumbar curvature pulls the pelvic organs back away from the lower front abdominal wall, over the pubic bones, where they belong. Prolapse isn't the pelvic organs falling down, they are falling back into the vaginal space. This is one reason why kegel exercises are of no value. The so-called pelvic floor is really a wall at the back of the pelvis, which is oriented like a ring on its edge, not like a basin with the opening at the bottom.

The Whole Woman approach is simple: Change the posture, change the prolapse.

This may seem overly simplistic, but I can assure you it is backed up with solid science. My book, *Saving the Whole Woman,** has almost 400 citations to books, research, and scholarly papers.

For the post-surgery woman (hysterectomy, mesh, bladder or uterine suspension, or other "repair"), results are less predictable. But many women who are struggling with post-surgery prolapse have benefited from my methods.

My point is this: prolapse is not a life sentence. In fact, you are the only one who can solve the problem. Relearning how you sit, stand, lift, and carry takes some time and effort. The payoff is regaining control of your health and the confidence that your body will continue to work well for you for years to come.

---

*Kent, *Saving the Whole Woman.*

◻ *Posture for Well-Being*

All women would do well to bring more awareness to their posture to support the body. Stand looking straight ahead, tucking your chin slightly down, relaxed, not rigid. Let your weight be distributed 50/50 on each leg. Standing off center greatly distorts posture. The knees should be slightly softened and not pushed right back. Stand with the inside of your feet parallel and hip-width apart. Any slight angling of the feet outward will make it more difficult to feel the lower body. Let your weight be equally distributed through the whole foot, not hanging heavily on the heels. Relax the pelvic floor, the vagina, and the anus. Then relax the belly fully. Lengthen your neck and then relax your shoulders. Lift and rotate your shoulders back in a circular motion. Then gently lift the rib cage, which creates an opening and more spaciousness in the solar plexus and diaphragm area. You will notice that this posture will slightly tilt your pelvis back, allowing the organs to sit more in their place. Stand

and be in this position, while synching to your inner body. Observe how bringing more awareness to your posture increases your inner cellular aliveness and sense of well-being. And most importantly it puts your body in a position that supports the pelvic organ alignment. This posture can be adapted for sitting as well, and can be helpful in the case of prolapse.

Posture Aids Blood Flow

This postural realignment creates a lifting action of the diaphragm that aids us twofold: (1) it aids realignment of the organs and pelvis as discussed, and (2) it allows for unobstructed blood flow to the whole lower abdominal region through the main aorta (oxygenated, arterial blood) and the vena cava (used, deoxygenated blood). This postural lifting action enables the flow of fresh oxygenated blood from the heart to the whole abdominal cavity (and the rest of the body), bathing and nourishing the tissues and organs with fresh, new red blood cells, nutrients, hormones, amino acids, oxygen, vitamins, minerals, plasma, and protein—flushing the organs and replenishing and nourishing the entire abdominal cavity. The used, deoxygenated blood is carried back to the chamber of the heart through the vena cava, via the lungs, where the blood is reoxygenated, and thus continues the flow.

This action gives the diaphragm and pelvic floor, similar in shape and structure, the opportunity to engage with each other. In unison they become like a pressurized cabin where everything sits better, providing a better chance of correct organ placement. Therefore, shallow breathing only in the upper chest will naturally constrict blood flow to the pelvic area, whereas diaphragmatic breathing, or deep breathing, is breathing that is done by contracting the diaphragm, a muscle located horizontally between the thoracic cavity and abdominal cavity. During this type of breathing the chest rises and the belly expands as air enters the lungs.

Lovemaking during Prolapse Condition

The devastation of having organ prolapse can pull a woman apart emotionally, as can all afflictions in this area, whether they are surgery, organ removal, ongoing infections, or something else. Like breast issues, they make a woman feel very vulnerable and she may question her ability to meet a man sexually ever again. Doubts about her body, shame at having the condition, and shutting down to protect herself can all affect her ability to open to any kind of sex, even conscious lovemaking.

But the heartening news is that lovemaking is still possible with prolapse. In fact the Making Love approach that we both endorse is magic for prolapse. Women have reported that the conscious, gentle approach, including soft, relaxed entry (see chapter 8), has been an absolute godsend to them. Lovemaking in this way will also bring more blood circulation to the area, which again is also very healing for the organs. When erection happens from a relaxed state within the vagina, this can in fact help to reposition the prolapse.

Maintaining flow of bowel function is imperative to reduce the symptoms of prolapse, and additionally so that lovemaking can be more easeful. It's important to void the bowel so that there is no bulk. A balanced diet that promotes ease of elimination is key. Some women use a magnesium supplement or high doses of vitamin C and probiotics. Ask your health practitioner to guide you. You may want to consider a series of cleansing treatments of the bowel through colonic irrigation if elimination is an issue and also for general health.

Castor Oil Packs

Castor oil is an age-old remedy for inflammation and constipation, to loosen toxins from the system and remove them. You can do a castor oil pack in any area that feels inflamed or stagnant, particularly the abdominal organs. Spread warmed, organic castor oil lavishly over the area, place a barrier such as plastic wrap over that, cover with a large towel, and tighten it around your belly. Then place a warm heat pack on top and rest for at least an hour lying down. It can take some organizing but it is worth it. You will find that your bowels may soften and move once again. It will make you stop and rest while nourishing and detoxifying. See a medical or alternative practitioner if the situation persists. It's important to make sure every day that there is "movement at the station," as an Australian might say, so that there is no buildup compromising your organs, preventing further complications.

The journey to wholeness as woman is not only healing past hurts, both emotional and physical scars, but to remember that the body is designed naturally to uplift, enliven, and bring joy.

The woman sharing this story discovered both the Making Love approach and the Whole Woman work by Christine Kent at around the same time:

Because I felt so vulnerable physically, I just didn't want to make love the way we had done in the past. I didn't feel like being intimate at all because I felt being in certain positions made me vulnerable. I had a fear of fully relaxing because I wasn't sure if my organs would fall out. When I started to make love this way, I became aware of how much I was holding internally. I also completely stopped doing kegel exercises; they were not helping. I did five years of kegels fairly regularly, on and off, being very diligent with a physiotherapist coaching me. Literally within two weeks of the better posture and proper voiding, symptoms were almost gone. This, coinciding with making love in more relaxation and not being goal oriented, is so far removed from where we were. With the Making Love approach, I feel so much more accepting of my body than I did before. He is more accepting, maybe even more than I am, and it's all down to how we are connecting differently. We are so much more comfortable in our bodies, so the prolapse is now all part and parcel of it. There are positions that I avoid, any that cause tension, but even this doesn't feel like an issue anymore.

RELAX THE PELVIC FLOOR
WITH AWARENESS

The musculature of the pelvic floor, when tightened, pulls up like a parachute into a central knotty tendon that you can feel with your hand when you contract. A lump just between the vagina and the anus will become palpable under your touch. It is here in particular that our tensions accumulate, spreading down and affecting the energy and structure of the legs and feet. We are continually pulling up the floor of the abdomen. Any time you put your awareness in your pelvic floor you will discover that it is tight, and when you relax and release the tissues, the musculature may drop down an inch!

The prime characteristic of the pelvic floor is that we are always clenching it, pulled up and contracted, and are basically unconscious of this central tension. Since I [Diana] discovered my pelvic floor a few decades ago, it has been a constant reference point for me. I started taking my awareness to my pelvic floor and I would find I was holding it tense *every* time. I would consciously release it, my body would take a huge sigh of relief, my shoulders would relax, and I would feel immediately more at ease, with my legs and feet more in contact with the earth. Moments or minutes later when I would inwardly revisit this spot, I would find that it was again slightly tight! Regardless of how many times I consciously let go and relaxed, the second my awareness was absent and I went into switch-off mode, there was always a pull upward to create a subtle tightening. Every time you remember it is an act of presence, and you are inviting relaxation and expansion within your body.

Toning through Awareness

Many women fear relaxing the pelvic floor because of a fear of a loss of strength and tone. However, when the pelvic floor is constantly under a subtle tension, this is not healthy for the tissues and pelvic integrity. Just bringing this part of your body to your awareness can make a big difference. Here is a small exercise that can tone the area, making it more resilient.

◑ Toning the Pelvic Floor

First identify the pelvic floor while standing. Pull up all the muscles around your genitals and anus, as if you are attempting to stop the flow of urine. It's easy. Squeeze a little tighter and exaggerate the tightness. Contract the musculature, and then let it go, relax and widen. Imagine that you are bottoming out, emptying out through the vagina and anus. Let the aliveness spread down the legs. If you can, feel the new inner sensations that come with this.

Practice these contractions and relaxations a few times to get the sense of relaxation and how it feels in the pelvic floor. And then feel welcome to relax your pelvic floor as often as possible, and wherever you are. Basically you can relax anywhere and any time (with or without the contraction phase), while waiting in line, chatting at a cocktail party, sitting in a car . . . it's okay, nobody can see what's going on and it feels delightful. And you can also repeatedly relax the pelvic floor (and thereby the vagina) when making love. Suddenly you will find yourself more at ease, more secure, and able to flow with the moment.

Make this pelvic-floor relaxation an awareness exercise that you do repeatedly all day long for years on end, because it delivers vitality and more consciousness to the genital area. But it's important not to do the contraction-and-relaxation sequence mechanically or unconsciously, otherwise you miss the point and ultimately this lack of awareness will make the vagina tougher and less sensitive and receptive.

Understand instead that you are keeping your pelvic floor toned and there is a need to balance the pulling up phase with the releasing down phase, and doing so slowly, millimeter by millimeter, you will observe how the consciousness in the area grows. Many women find it easier to try this while lying down. You can contract to the count of five (or seven) as you breathe in, and then relax to the same count as you exhale. Also reverse the breathing from time to time, so that you relax as you breathe in and contract when you exhale. This reversed breathing of contracting when you breathe out has been found to be very beneficial for women with prolapse.

The beauty of awareness is that it knows no bounds. Women can always find another layer of perception in the vagina by focusing the awareness into the vagina and asking, *Can I be more open? Can I be more receptive?* Miraculously the tissues will widen a few millimeters, getting fuller as the very cells are penetrated with consciousness, and on occasion, if you are making love, the male penis may respond with jerking movements, snaking more deeply into the vagina.

Tonus, Not Tension

In my retreats I (Diana) have always, since the beginning, encouraged participants to widen and relax the pelvic floor and vagina. However sometimes I am asked if relaxing is really the right thing to do, as the general understanding is that we need to have more strength and holding in that area, especially as some women suffer incontinence or prolapse of different kinds. Yes, it is definitely true that the area needs to be resilient, however it is tonus (constant low-level activity) that is required, not the adding of tension to already existing unconscious tensions. With the area already contracted, we add tension to tension through mechanical strengthening practices, and ultimately we are not serving ourselves.

The way forward is to instill the area with relaxation and subtle life force, and with that level as the foundation, to consciously contract and relax, and thus increase the tonus and vitality of the tissues in the area. So-called pelvic-floor trainings have become quite popular in some countries, where people intensely focus on strengthening the pelvic floor over a series of weekends. However, we have had reports from women who suffered from severe cystitis and bladder inflammations as a result, due, in my opinion, to adding too much tension to an already tense area (and one that is usually completely out of our awareness). And importantly, the procedure is generally done mechanically and without the balancing and regenerating effects of awareness, softening, relaxing, and widening.

As we have said before, every woman is different and what works for one may not work for another. Keep exploring, like the intrepid traveler of the world of your body. Trust it. Experiment with how these exercises feel. The important thing is that whatever works for you, practice it daily; bring it into your awareness on an ongoing basis. This will support your body indefinitely on many levels.

It is often through the suffering that women endure through our bodies—through the many experiences of just being a woman (menstruation, childbirth, menopause, illness, difficulties). Such experiences can be vital crossroads on our journey to wholeness. We can begin to heal an inner part of our femininity, and perhaps even our lineage of being female. Seeing the gift in the challenge will bring us more *into* our bodies, into the truth of who we are. It actually compels us to be connected to our bodies. It is a wakeup call from the soul to nurture, self-care, heal, and embrace the journey of woman with love and understanding. Rather than seeing your body as something that has betrayed you, see your body as your trusted companion in this life and treat it generously as you would treat a dear friend—with compassion, love, and friendliness.

DAILY PELVIC SELF-CARE

You can see how important it is for women to at least be aware of how to care for themselves and their pelvic organs, through self-massage of the belly, attending to the bowels and elimination organs through good nutrition and regular daily exercise, and moving things through energetically. Any stagnation in your daily life will cause stagnation in your body. We are hardwired that way. It is important to just bring this part of the body into awareness while doing your daily activities. Yoga, walking, swimming, and belly dancing are all wonderful ways to support your body and pelvic organs. Seek out a yoga teacher who is particularly interested and versed in issues of the female body.

It is little surprise that traditional dancers in the indigenous cultures of the world rhythmically beat through their feet and move deeply from the hips, unafraid and untamed through their lower bodies. This is true wildness, and Western women could do well to follow this wisdom to bring them out of the wilderness of these lost territories of our bodies to become fully embodied.

ひ Pelvic Rocking

Lie on a flat, firm cushioned surface such as a yoga mat or rug. Visualize the location of your womb in the center of your lower pelvis (see location in fig. 11.1 on page 167). Place your hands over the area if that feels good. Lie still and breathe in and out naturally.

Lift your knees with your feet flat on the floor and close your eyes. Begin a slow rock of your pelvis forward and back by first tipping the pelvis backward and arching your back, then curling it forward and rounding your back. You will notice that if you allow your body to follow this tipping and tucking without restriction that as you tip your pelvis back it will create an arching of your back and an opening of your chest with an expansion of your belly. Then rock the pelvis forward so that your tailbone curls forward and your spine and back are flattening on the floor, belly gently sunken toward your spine.

Then invite your breath to synchronize with the movement. Breathe in while you are tilting back, and breathe out while you are tucking your tailbone under. As you do, bring your awareness to your breasts and heart opening. You can start to create a slow rhythm, and it is wonderful for womb awareness and connecting the breasts and heart with the womb. And remember—always in relaxation! Consciously relaxing the vagina, continue to rock forward and back. The relaxation sounds like a contradiction but it changes the quality of your experience.

Do this for a few minutes and then relax. Then try again for another few minutes, then relax. Rest once you're done and go inward with your awareness to notice the aftereffects of the exercise. You may even feel the inner rod of magnetism as you rest. Allow the energy to spread through your body, visualizing it going to your fingertips and toes.

⊙ Womb Awareness and Grounding

As much as possible, momentarily remind yourself to stand, walk, and sit with postural alignment. Avoid slouching and slumping. Once you start to bring more awareness to this part of your body, you can use womb awareness to ground yourself. This can be used if you feel yourself a little emotionally off balance or even going into a conversation with your partner that you feel may be challenging. Standing still, imagine that you are sending roots from your hips down through both of your legs and into the earth. Close your eyes. Go inward and visualize the location of your womb, tucked in between the front and back of your lower pelvis. You can even imagine a light or a symbol there. Begin walking consciously with womb awareness. You will find it brings you more peace, centeredness, and inner strength.*

⊙ The Healing Power of Walking

It is extremely helpful for all women, especially those with menopausal difficulties, to take a walk in nature as often as possible. It is understood that our female forebears walked between five and ten miles a day and our bodies are built for movement. A minimum of twenty minutes will start to increase serotonin levels, have an impact on your metabolism, your pelvic organs, your whole system, and your psychological state. Walking consciously with womb awareness is very grounding and holds you in the present. We suggest that you walk with relaxed, receptive vision. Menopause is a time when we want to nourish, replenish, and regenerate the body through appropriate exercise. Any exercise that you choose to do should be invigorating but not exhausting, as excessive strenuous exercise can drain the adrenals and result in depletion. Nature is showering us constantly with its splendor and healing vibrations and often we are not even aware of it, so walking consciously in nature is uplifting for the body and soul.

---

*Partly adapted from the teachings of Rachael Jayne Groover, author of *Powerful and Feminine: How to Increase Your Magnetic Presence and Attract the Attention you Want* (Fort Collins, Colo.: Deep Pacific Press, 2011).

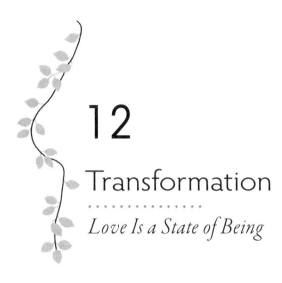

12

Transformation

Love Is a State of Being

Love is the radiance, the fragrance of knowing oneself, of being oneself. . . . Love is overflowing joy. Love is when you have seen who you are; then there is nothing left except to share your being with others. Love is when you have seen that you are not separate from existence. Love is when you have felt an organic, orgasmic unity with all that is. Love is not a relationship. Love is a state of being. It has nothing to do with anybody else. One is not in love; one is love. And of course when one is love, one is in love, but that is an outcome, a by-product; that is not the source. The source is that one is love.

Osho transcribed teachings,
The Guest: Talks on Kabir

A CALL TO LOVE

It's time. Time for women to make a stand for love. We need it. The world needs it. Domestic violence is escalating in our cities and towns all around the world. The world needs us to value ourselves and our bodies beyond our childbearing use, beyond fulfilling someone else's need or lust, to trust our bodies, and to be the light for other women

to challenge the conditioning set before us and make love our priority. When a woman values herself enough to embrace her true femininity, discovered through the innocence and purity of her own direct
experience (of her ecstatic nature) rather than an idealized, romanti-
cized interpretation of the feminine, she has the capacity to heal herself
and the collective, and to lead and inspire her children, her sisters, her
brothers, and her community. Women have a central place in the world
today: to lead with and through the heart.

Do not underestimate your role as menopausal woman. You are
in a very influential place in your family and community. No matter
what your current circumstances, valuing yourself and your position
as an elder with humility and grace, valuing the powerful needs of our
bodies to slow down and be nourished at this most important entry
into the wisdom years, will flow over into your life, your relationships,
and your love. As each woman heals and changes her consciousness
around sex and menopause, everyone around her is touched. It is up
to us, if we want to make a difference on this planet today, to step up
and empower ourselves through awareness, insight, and understanding, opening the door to love. The more love you give, the more love
you have. And that quality of giving has nothing to do with compromising oneself.

Love is our basic nature, and it is our most powerful resource. We
must harness the feminine through our love. But for that to happen we
must be willing to meet our own barriers to love and pleasure within
our bodies. We must not be miserly with our love and let our toxic
emotions rule and enclose our hearts. The world needs the very thing
that we are most natural at giving—and that is this quality of love.
Nurturing and growing our awareness is how we show up as women,
how we relate to our own bodies, and how we show up in lovemaking.
But remember this must be done from a full cup and not a half-empty
cup. The way we move through our elder years will bring us true fulfillment and bring more joy and meaning to our lives. We can pave the way
for younger and younger women, our daughters, our granddaughters,

giving them permission as well to trust their bodies and inner beings, especially in the realm of sexuality.

MAKE TIME FOR LOVE

One of the strong suggestions we make is for couples to make the time for love and then actually show up for the making-love date. Because we have been so programmed to expect less-than-satisfying experiences from lovemaking, the common scenario at any age is to make everything else more important before getting around to loving. Knowing beforehand that you will make love can be perceived as removing the spontaneity; however, when you intentionally choose to create space and time for love, you will arrive more present and inwardly prepared. Countless couples over the years have attested to the value of this, and of course, this is our own experience as well.

If you have a partner, set aside time for loving once a week or twice a week. It can be very relaxing for a man when he knows that the time has been set. Otherwise he is wondering when the next chance at intimacy will come around, when his woman will "let him in," and this can cause unnecessary tension, arguments, and emotions. If you still have children at home, try to make it at a time during the day when they are not there. Be creative. And if you are a woman on your own, set aside a time for tuning in to your body and doing the breast meditation, for instance, or any of the exercises in the book. The regularity and repetition of the practices gives rise to the inner transformation, the radiance and sweetness of the feminine.

RESISTANCE TO INTIMACY

If you feel resistance it's still good to just show up and be present. Your man will appreciate you just because of that. It means a lot to him to know that you want to participate as well. If there is resistance, simply and lovingly say so. However, as mentioned earlier, it is important to understand that resistance is *usually the resistance to being present per se,* not necessarily a resistance to intimacy or to sex itself. Remember that your body requires time to warm up and with that process, resistance will melt away. Also the body is always happy to make love and mostly it is the mind that is not happy about it, so the way forward is to be present within yourself, to come home to you first and be guided by your body, rather than led by your mind. If you are married or in a committed relationship, it is also interesting to look at the reasons you *choose not to have sex,* as power plays can emerge in the withholding from a loved one. When faced with making a choice, notice whether you are honoring your pride, your ego, or your body and spirit.

Making Love Is Not Only Penetration

It's helpful to broaden the definition of making love. It definitely does not *only* mean penis in vagina. Just two bodies lying together in awareness generates love. Usually when a woman simply lies like this and relaxes into her own being, she may eventually feel a yes emerging from her body. Woman carries such a pressure inside her, so anything she can do to consciously and inwardly relax will help.

Getting into the practice of intentionally creating space in your schedule will invite more possibilities and opportunities. Create the space to relax, enter into your bodies, and awaken the aliveness via your dynamic poles—women nipples, men perineum—and allow love to flow. If you don't have a partner then still set aside times to be with yourself and your inner world, and this act of self-love will bring tremendous fulfillment.

Communicate Where You Are At

If it is really not the moment for you to make love, then communicate your reasons and feelings from your heart. Anything communicated from the heart will usually be received by the heart of the other person. And the most important thing to watch is that you are not getting emotional yourself and being a little bit aggressive or blaming.

One woman shares that her husband has softened so much toward her, now that she has made the weekly commitment and time for loving:

He appreciates the fact that I show up even if I don't feel like showing up. We start with an intention and check in with each other. There is anxiety every time, every single time for me. For him, every single time, he is excited to be there! We check in and I cry and get through it pretty quickly. I feel there is a much healthier connection now. Now I feel okay to say where I am at about making love in the evening (which doesn't work for me), whereas before I would have pushed through, outwardly performed but shut down on the inside. As soon as we get together and the candles are lit, he is erect straight away. Before, I felt pressured to even touch his erect penis. I felt I had to do something with it, to perform, to please. Now we are both so comfortable with IT being there.

Love exists at our very source. When a woman becomes attuned to the love inside herself first and foremost, when she turns her attention inward, there is no question of being loved or being loving—they become one. No longer does she need to seek out another for love. And no longer does she need to actively give in order to receive love. She simply is. She is love. You are love. It's that simple. Woman is extremely magnetic and radiant when she simply embodies the power within, rather than trying to have power *over* another.

Innocence and freshness return when you become aware that you are love and that your body is love itself. This merging with the Divine, with God, with "the oneness" is like merging with the ultimate lover, the ultimate intimate beloved. Virtually every soul, heart, and body longs for this sense of union and dissolving. Being able to merge energetically with yourself, alone or with another person, gives you the opportunity to meet the Divine. A relaxed woman is pure love, a gift to herself, her relationship, and her family, and a force so needed in our world.

When we know, understand, and appreciate that love is a state of being, we see that it is the intrinsic spiritual quality of each woman. Then we are ready to give up the social stagnation and feeling invisible and discarded through ignorance. Instead we support the evolution of womanhood (and thus of manhood) at this rich and important time in history. Through valuing our beautiful bodies, no matter what shape or size, appreciating and understanding the blessing of being a woman helps us embrace the powerful gift of this courageous time of our lives—menopause.

With all our hearts, we wish you an inspiring grand walk into the second spring of your life! Together we are strong as each individual woman weaves her special thread into the tapestry of consciousness. May you blaze the trail for the women to come, and in honor of those women in whose valiant footsteps we follow.

Recommended Books
and Resources

WE HAVE FOUND THE FOLLOWING BOOKS and resources to be extremely helpful and inspirational, particularly regarding hormones, facts about the female body, and therapeutic options. Please note that some titles express a different view on sex from the approach we have proposed in this book.

BOOKS

Arvigo Practitioners. *Journeys into Healing: Inspiring Experiences of Arvigo Practitioners and Their Clients.* Antrim, N.H.: The Arvigo Institute, 2014.

Bays, Brandon. *The Journey: An Extraordinary Guide for Healing Yourself and Setting Yourself Free.* New York: Harper Collins, 2012.

Groover, Rachael Jayne. *Powerful and Feminine: How to Increase Your Magnetic Presence and Attract the Attention You Want.* Fort Collins, Colo.: Deep Pacific Press, 2011.

Hertoghe, Thierry, M.D. *The Hormone Solution: Stay Younger Longer with Natural Hormone and Nutrition Therapies.* New York: Three Rivers Press, 2002.

Kent, Christine Ann. *Saving the Whole Woman: Natural Alternatives to Surgery for Pelvic Organ Prolapse and Urinary Incontinence.* 2nd ed. Albuquerque, N.M.: Bridgeworks Inc., 2008.

Kenton, Leslie. *Passage to Power: Natural Menopause Revolution.* London: Random House, 1995.

Lassiter, Judith. *The Woman's Book of Yoga and Health: A Lifelong Guide to Wellness.* Boston: Shambhala, 2002.

Lee, John R., M.D., with Virginia Hopkins. *What Your Doctor May Not Tell You about Menopause: The Breakthrough Book on* Natural *Hormone Balance.* New York: Grand Central Publishing/Hachette, 2004.

Long, Barry. *Making Love: Sexual Love the Divine Way.* London: Barry Long Books, 2006.

———. *To Woman in Love: A Book of Letters.* London: Barry Long Books, 1995.

Northrup, Christiane, M.D. *Women's Bodies, Women's Wisdom: Creating Physical and Emotional Health and Healing.* Rev. ed. New York: Bantam Books, 2010.

———. *The Wisdom of Menopause: Creating Physical and Emotional Health during the Change.* New York: Bantam Books, 2012.

Osho. *Sex Matters: From Sex to Superconsciousness.* New York: St. Martin's Press, 2003.

———. *The Book of Secrets.* New York: St. Martin's Press, 1998.

Pert, Candace B., Ph.D. *Molecules of Emotion: The Science behind Mind-Body Medicine.* New York: Simon & Schuster, 1999.

Richardson, Diana. *Slow Sex: A Path to Fulfilling and Sustainable Sexuality.* Rochester, Vt.: Destiny Books, 2011.

———. *Tantric Love Letters: A Collection of Experiences, Questions, and Answers.* Arlesford, Hants, U.K.: "O" Books, 2011.

———. *Tantric Orgasm for Women.* Rochester, Vt.: Destiny Books, 2004.

———. *The Heart of Tantric Sex: A Unique Guide to Love and Sexual Fulfillment.* Arlesford, Hants, U.K.: "O" Books, 2002.

Richardson, Diana, and Michael Richardson. *Tantric Love: Feeling versus Emotion—Golden Rules to Make Love Easy.* Arlesford, Hants, U.K.: "O" Books, 2010.

———. *Tantric Sex for Men: Making Love a Meditation.* Rochester, Vt.: Destiny Books, 2010.

Robinson, Marnia. *Cupid's Poisoned Arrow: From Habit to Harmony in Sexual Relationships.* Berkeley, Calif.: North Atlantic Books, 2009.

Rosenberg, Marshall. *Nonviolent Communication: A Language of Life.* 3rd ed. Encinitas, Calif.: PuddleDancer Press, 2015.

Siegel, Dan. *The Whole-Brain Child: 12 Revolutionary Strategies to Nurture Your Child's Developing Mind.* New York: Bantam, 2012.

Turton, Sharon. *The Art of Peaceful Parenting: Seven Steps to Connecting with Your Child.* Glebe, NSW, Australia: Atlantis Books, 2016.

Weed, Susun S. *New Menopausal Years: The Wise Woman Way.* Woodstock, N.Y.: Ashtree Publishing, 2002.

Wilson, Gary. *Your Brain on Porn: Internet Pornography and the Emerging Science of Addiction.* Margate, Kent, U.K.: Commonwealth Publishing, 2015.

AUDIO AND VIDEO

Richardson, Diana. *Slow Sex: How Sex Makes You Happy—A New Style of Loving* (DVD). Cologne, Germany: Innenwelt Verlag, 2011. Order at amazon.co.uk (note English and German tracks on the same DVD). For English download only go to www.einfach-liebe-shop.de.

Richardson, Diana, and Michael Richardson. *Ma Lua Light Meditation for Women.* Guided breast meditation CD with music. (English and German tracks available on the same CD.) Cologne, Germany: Innenwelt Verlag, 2009. Order at www.amazon.co.uk.

RESOURCES

Websites

www.theartoffemininepresence.com
www.arvigotherapy.com
www.healthywomen.org
www.beautifulcervix.com
www.mayanhealing.com.au
www.menopause.org
www.progesteronetherapy.com
www.wholewoman.com

Women's Retreats

Diana and Janet offer five-day women's retreats in Switzerland and Australia, respectively.

Switzerland: Diana Puja Richardson, www.livinglove.com

Australia: Janet McGeever, www.janetmcgeever.com

The Making Love Retreat

Making Love, a seven-day Tantra meditation retreat for couples designed by Diana and Michael Richardson, www.livinglove.com and www.loveforcouples.com

Authorized Teachers of the Making Love Retreat

- Australia: www.makingloveretreat.com.au
- Germany: www.paarweise.info
- France: www.amourenconscience.ch
- Spain and Italy: www.isabellamagdala.com and www.making loveretreat.es
- Switzerland, www.livinglove.com or www.love4couples.com

About the Authors

Diana Richardson is known as the pioneer of the Slow Sex movement and, along with her partner, Michael Richardson, is the creator of the life-changing weeklong Making Love Retreat, which they have been offering since 1995. A massage therapist and bodyworker for thirty-five years, Diana was born in South Africa, where she completed her Law degree. She lived in India for many years, where she began her research and inquiry into the union of sex and meditation in 1985. This is her eighth book on the tantric approach to love and sex. She is now based in Switzerland with Michael, where they continue to guide couples in the art of slow, conscious sex.

For more information about their work, please visit their websites:
www.livinglove.com or **www.love4couples.com**
Contact email: info@livinglove.com

Janet McGeever is an Australian-born writer who has been a practicing psychotherapist since 1999. A speaker at Noosa TEDx in 2013, she has been a facilitator of women's work for over twenty years and has held couples retreats since 2009. An authorized facilitator in Australia since 2012 of the Richardsons' transformational Making Love Retreats for couples, she began her career as an art teacher, eventually moving to body-based psychotherapy. Holding a master's degree in experiential and creative arts therapy, she is the creator of "Womantime—Ancient Wisdom for the Modern Day Woman," a retreat and feminine self-care teaching for women of all ages, which evolved out of the writing of this book.

For more information about her work, please visit her websites:
www.janetmcgeever.com and **www.makingloveretreat.com.au**
Contact email: info@janetmcgeever.com

BOOKS OF RELATED INTEREST

Tantric Orgasm for Women
by Diana Richardson

Tantric Sex for Men
Making Love a Meditation
by Diana Richardson and Michael Richardson

Slow Sex
The Path to Fulfilling and Sustainable Sexuality
by Diana Richardson

The Complete Illustrated Kama Sutra
Edited by Lance Dane

Yoni Massage
Awakening Female Sexual Energy
by Michaela Riedl

Tao Tantric Arts for Women
Cultivating Sexual Energy, Love, and Spirit
by Minke de Vos
Foreword by Mantak Chia

Healing Love through the Tao
Cultivating Female Sexual Energy
by Mantak Chia

The Sexual Practices of Quodoushka
Teachings from the Nagual Tradition
by Amara Charles

INNER TRADITIONS • BEAR & COMPANY
P.O. Box 388
Rochester, VT 05767
1-800-246-8648
www.InnerTraditions.com

Or contact your local bookseller